R.W. Dal Negro · L. Allegra (Eds)

Pneumological Aspects of Gastroesophageal Reflux

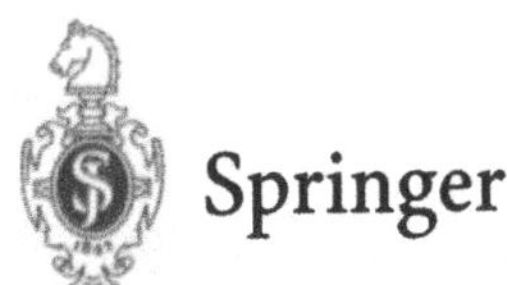

Springer

ROBERTO WALTER DAL NEGRO
Lung Department
Bussolengo General Hospital
Bussolengo (Verona), Italy

LUIGI ALLEGRA
Institute of Respiratory Diseases
University of Milan
IRCCS Ospedale Maggiore
Milan, Italy

The Editors and Authors wish to thank **Astra Farmaceutici S.p.A.** for the support and help in the realization of this volume

---

© Springer-Verlag Italia,1999
Originally published by Springer-Verlag Italia,Milano in 1999

ISBN 978-88-470-0049-0

Library of Congress Cataloging-in-Publication Data: Pneumological aspects of gastroesophageal reflux / R.W. Dal Negro, L. Allegra (eds). p. cm. Includes bibliographical references and index.
ISBN 978-88-470-0049-0   ISBN 978-88-470-2147-1 (eBook)
DOI 10.1007/978-88-470-2147-1
Gastroesophageal reflux. 2. Gastroesophageal reflux-
Complications. 3. Asthma. 4. Bronchi--Diseases. I. Dal Negro, Roberto. [DNLM: 1. Gastroesophageal Reflux--complications. 2. Gastroesophageal Reflux--physiopathology. 3. Bronchial Diseases-etiology. 4. Bronchoconstriction. 5. Gastroesophageal Reflux-therapy. 6. Lung Diseases--etiology. WI 250 P738 1999] RC815.7.P64 1999 616,3'2--dc21 DNLM/DLC for Library of Congress 99-24353 CIP

Cover design: Simona Colombo, Milan
Typesetting and layout: Graphostudio, Milan

SPIN: 10715380

Preface

There is a growing body of evidence suggesting that gastroesophageal reflux may be involved in the development, persistence or aggravation of different respiratory diseases. Unfortunately, the recognition of the cause-effect relationship between gastroesophageal reflux and pulmonary disorders is difficult to establish, and pharmacologic correction of the reflux is not always associated with improvement of the respiratory symptoms. This new book entitled *Pneumological Aspects of Gastroesophageal Reflux* and edited by Roberto Dal Negro and Luigi Allegra covers this intriguing relation between gastroesophageal reflux and respiratory diseases, mainly aspiration pneumonia and asthma, but also interstitial lung diseases and chronic obstructive pulmonary disease (COPD). The contributors, all Italian, have solid personal experience in the issues discussed, and this experience is reflected in the content of the chapters. Indeed, the book is easy to read, appealing, and full of useful, practical information. All aspects of gastroesophageal reflux are discussed. After the chapters devoted to epidemiology, basic physiology, pharmacology, and clinical manifestations, the book includes interesting and useful chapters on diagnosis and treatment. These chapters correctly emphasize how difficult it is to establish in an individual patient the relationship between gastroesophageal reflux and pulmonary disorder, and how carefully the patient has to be followed to monitor the response to treatment. This book is a useful reference not only for pulmonologists, but also for gastroenterologists and internists.

Antonino Mistretta
Professor of Pneumology
University of Catania

Leonardo M. Fabbri
Director, The Research Center
on Asthma and COPD
University of Ferrara

Table of Contents

Diagnostic Techniques for Gastroesophageal Reflux Detection

Diagnostic Techniques for Assessing Pulmonary Involvement

Therapy

Gastroesophageal Reflux in Gastroenterology

Epidemiology of Gastroesophageal Reflux

E. IERARDI[1], A. AMORUSO[1], R. FRANCAVILLA[2], D. ANNOSCIA[1], and A. FRANCAVILLA[1]

Introduction

Epidemiology investigates frequency, causes and distribution of a disease in a population from a specific geographic area to detect whether environment plays a role in health-related problems. The frequency of a disorder is evaluated by two parameters:

1. Incidence: number of new cases per 100 000 inhabitants per year;
2. Prevalence: percentage of cases in an examined population.

Gastroesophageal reflux (GER) is a condition characterised by the presence of a constant feature, e.g. reflux of gastric juice into the oesophagus, and inconstant aspects (not always observed), e.g. clinical symptoms or oesophagitis.

Epidemiological Evaluation of GER

Kitchin and Castell [1] represented GER as an "iceberg" that consisted of:

1. An emerging small portion, characterised by subjects undergoing specific tests for a diagnosis of GER because of the presence of important clinical signs;
2. A submerged large portion, represented by patients whose symptoms are not so marked to induce them to investigate a possible cause of the discomfort.

This definition clearly points out the limits of performing a correct epidemiological evaluation of GER. On the other hand, continuous 24-hour monitoring of oesophageal pH represents the gold standard to diagnose GER [2], even though studies with this technique cannot be performed on a large number of subjects. Moreover, there is not yet an agreement about normal ranges for a clear separation between "physiologic" and "pathologic" refluxes. In fact,

Departments of [1]Gastroenterology and [2]Paediatrics, University of Bari, Italy although most authors believe that a reflux index < 5% is likely to be normal and an index > 10% should be considered as pathologic, a value between 5% and 10% constitutes a grey zone requiring a more detailed evaluation [3].

The easiest method for an epidemiological evaluation of GER is the study of the prevalence of its symptoms in a population. Nevertheless, an unresolved problem in the epidemiology of gastrointestinal (GI) symptoms is represented by a marked overlap of chronic upper and lower GI complaints [4]. The concept that different functional GI disorders are the end result of a common set of pathophysiological disturbances has been suggested and the term "irritable gut" proposed [5]. In fact, 51% of patients with GER also suffer from irritable bowel syndrome [6]. Moreover, the role of delayed gastric emptying in the pathogenesis of GER is well known. Recently, a prospective study has shown that in 40%-50% of patients with GER, gastric functional problems are documented (antro-duodenal altered motility) [7]. Further problems related to clinical evaluation of GER are represented by its association and uncertain relationship with some conditions such as pregnancy [8], cholecystectomy [9] or *Helicobacter pylori* [10], as well as the possibility of extra-digestive signs which mask the characteristic clinical appearances [11-13].

GER symptoms may be described as chronic dyspepsia when this condition is defined as a recurrent or chronic pain or discomfort localised in the upper abdomen and lasting for 3 or more months [14]. In addition, dyspepsia subgroups have been identified in 1991 by a group of experts (Rome criteria):
1. *Ulcer-like*: well-localised pain in the epigastrium, relieved by food or anti-acids, occurring before meals, when hungry or at night, and showing a recurrent pattern.
2. *Dismotility-like*: early satiety, post-prandial fullness, nausea, retching and/or vomiting, bloating, and pain and/or discomfort aggravated by food.
3. *Reflux-like*: dyspepsia plus heartburn and/or acid regurgitation at least once a week.

On the other hand, peculiar GER symptoms (heartburn and acid regurgitation) may be observed even without other dyspeptic signs (symptomatic reflux). A recent report of Locke et al. [15] on the prevalence and clinical spectrum of GER symptoms in a sample of 2200 subjects aged 25-75 years from Olmsted County, Minnesota, showed that heartburn and acid regurgitation are present in more than 50% of the general population even if they are constant in less than 20%. Moreover, these typical signs are significantly associated with chest pain (23.1%), dysphagia (13.1%), globus sensation (7%), and asthma (9.3%).

Recently, Talley et al. attempted by factor analysis to identify natural groupings of upper and lower GI symptoms [16]. Results suggest that these symptoms fall into seven distinct groups. One of these is symptomatic GER. This study confirms that epidemiological evaluation of GER, based on the frequency of its clinical peculiarities, is able to reveal this condition only in the patients showing symptomatic reflux.

Another way to perform an epidemiological evaluation of GER is represented by the study of its most important consequence, i.e. oesophagitis. This method requires an endoscopic examination of the upper GI tract and therefore is limited to the patients undergoing this investigation.

Epidemiology of GER Symptoms

In 1976 Nebel et al. reported in a population of hospital employees that heartburn was present daily in 7%, weekly in 14% and monthly in 15% [17]. Daily values were meanly doubled when the study also involved hospitalised patients until reaching 25% in pregnant women [17]. These data are, on the whole, reflected by more recent ones of 1990 from Talley et al. [18]. In fact, these authors have described in Australia a daily, weekly and monthly prevalence of heartburn in dyspeptics of 7%, 13% and 24%, respectively [18].

Figure 1 reports the values of prevalence of GER symptoms observed in different studies performed in USA and Scandinavia in the decade 1981-1991. Results are different in relation to some variables such as the age of subjects and the recurrence of symptoms (daily, weekly, monthly). Nevertheless, a prevalence ranging from 5% to 15% in the adult population may be argued [19-21].

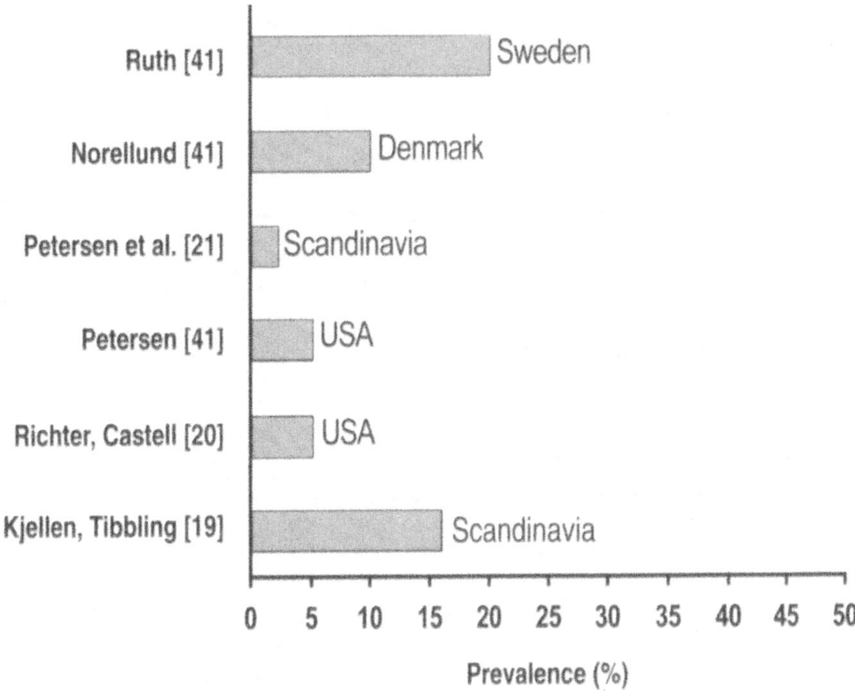

Fig. 1. Prevalence of GER symptoms in USA and Scandinavia in the ten-year period 1981-1991

Epidemiology of Oesophagitis

A value of 4.5 for the incidence of oesophagitis was reported by Rex et al. in a study performed in 1961 [22]. This datum has, of course, only historical importance. Ollyo et al. [23] studied this parameter in Switzerland in the same geographic area in 1963 and 1980, obtaining marked differences in the results: 10 and 138, respectively. These findings clearly suggest how the time of a study may significantly affect its result. Nevertheless, a value of 120, similar to the one found by Ollyo et al. in 1988, has been reported by Loof et al. [24] from the area of Uppsala, Sweden in the period 1988-1990.

More detailed data are available about the prevalence of oesophagitis since this parameter may be easily detected in centers in which a conspicuous number of upper endoscopic examinations are performed. Nevertheless, the results may differ as they are affected by many variables. This concept is apparent from Fig. 2 in which data are reported from a number of relevant studies performed in the twenty-year period from 1971 to 1991 [25-37]. Figure 3 illustrates the prevalence of oesophagitis in 3 countries (Italy, France and England) with similar social and economic conditions in the same period (1985-1988). Values markedly differ and are inversely related to the number of patients examined by

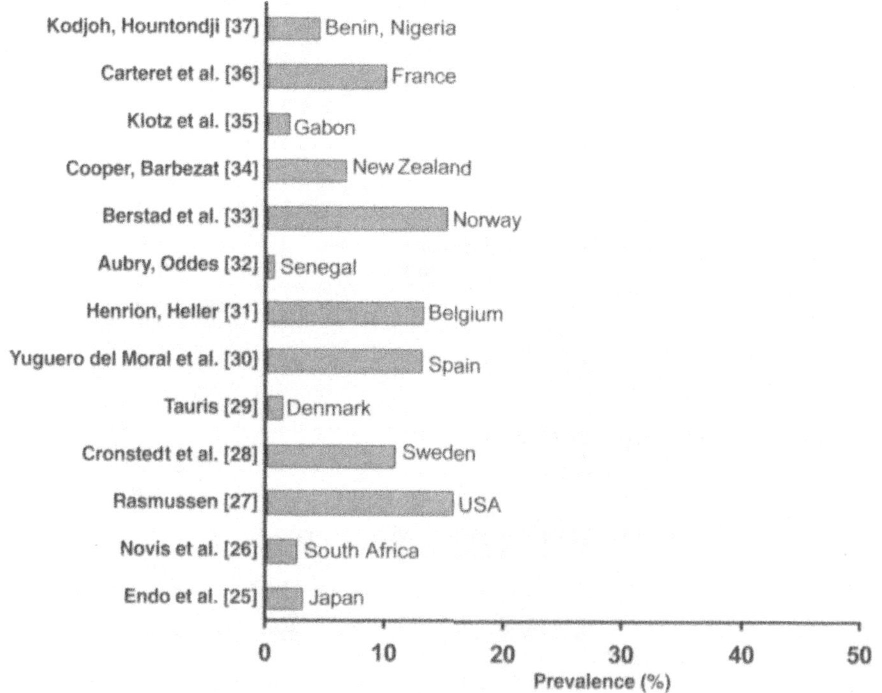

Fig. 2. Prevalence of oesophagitis in different geographic areas in the twenty-year period 1971-1991

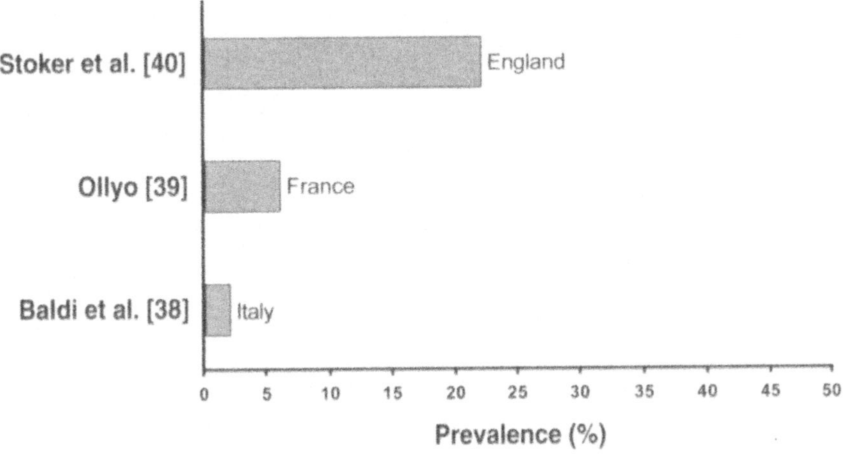

Fig. 3. Prevalence of oesophagitis from 3 countries (England, France and Italy) evaluated in the period 1985-1988

oesophagogastroduodenoscopy [38-40]. A possible explanation may be that the examination of a larger number of patients involves multiple centres, thereby increasing the intra-observer differences – known variables affecting studies based on the detection of anatomic alterations. On the other hand, while the Italian prevalence of oesophagitis described by Baldi et al. [38] in 1985 was 2.5%, in the value (8.6%) reported in a successive study by GISMAD in 1992-1993 on a similar total number of subjects [41] was significantly different. Thus, the period of study performance may possibly affect the results. This issue is raised even by the data from our centre (Department of Gastroenterology, University of Bari, Italy), as reported in Fig. 4. The prevalence of oesophagitis progressively increases every year in the period 1995-1997. This cannot be simply explained by the different times of examination nor by the intra-observer differences, since the periods are closer and endoscopic examinations are always performed by the same operators. Therefore, another variable needs to be considered such as the more accurate selection of patients undergoing endoscopy. This may be the consequence of having more detailed information. Finally, the data illustrated in Figs. 5 and 6, which concern a very large sample of patients, clearly show that oesophagitis prevalence in Italians is similar to that of duodenal ulcer and is markedly higher than that of gastric ulcer [41]. The same study demonstrated that 5%-10% of patients with oesophagitis show further complications (i.e. columnar cell metaplasia, Barrett's syndrome). Moreover, no difference has been observed among different geographic areas (northern, southern, central Italy and the islands).

In conclusion, epidemiological evidence of oesophagitis clearly demonstrates that some variables may significantly affect the data:
1. Period of the study
2. Intra-observer variations

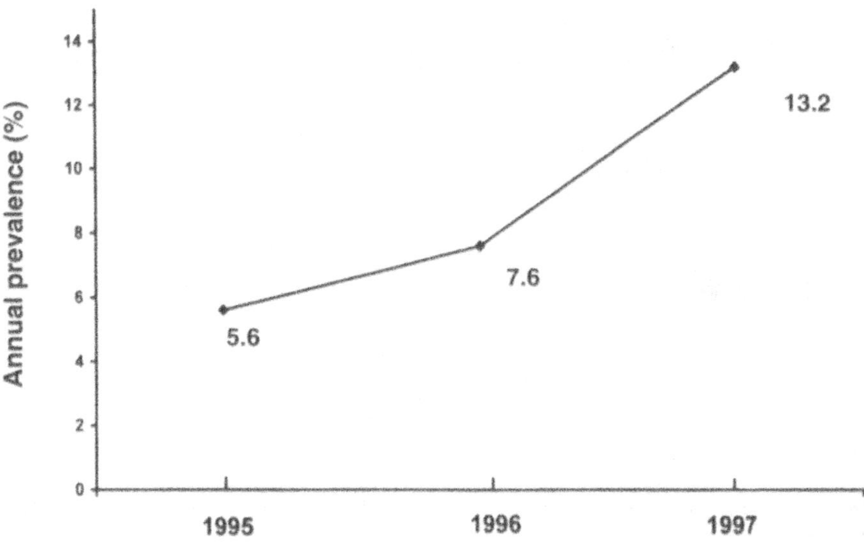

Fig. 4. Annual prevalence of oesophagitis in the three years 1995-1997 observed by the Gastroenterology Department of the University of Bari, Italy

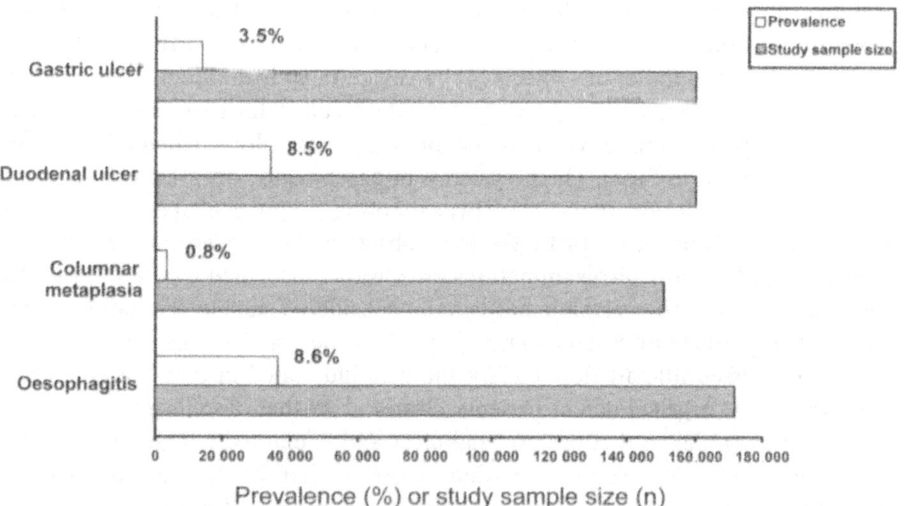

Fig. 5. Multicentre epidemiological data from the Italian Group for the Study of Digestive Motility, 1992-1993. Prevalence of gastric ulcer, duodenal ulcer, columnar metaplasia, and oesophagitis

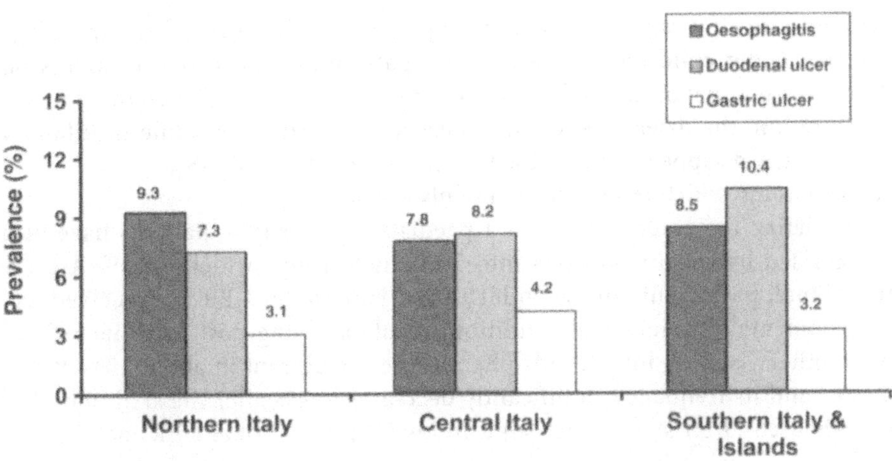

Fig. 6. Multicentre epidemiological data from the Italian Group for the Study of Digestive Motility, 1992-1993, referred to the different geographic areas of Italy

3. Number of subjects who are examined
4. Number of centres involved in the study
5. Selection of patients undergoing examination.

Despite the possibile variable results from epidemiological parameters, GER and its main anatomic consequence (oesophagitis) in particular are widely diffused in the general population and therefore constitute an important health-related problem.

Quality of Life in Patients with GER

Since GER is a common condition, some studies have examined the impact of this disease on the quality of life of patients. Cross-sectional studies have shown that psychological well-being scores of patients with untreated oesophagitis were similar to those of patients with untreated duodenal ulcer [42]. Successively in randomised placebo-controlled trials, GER treatment resulted in significant improvements in psychological and emotional well-being parameters such as sleep, role limitations, social functions and mental health [43, 44]. Moreover, patients with GER have more pain-related problems than those with other chronic diseases such as diabetes and hypertension [45]. Velanovich and Karmy-Jones [46] demonstrated that lower esophageal sphincter pressure is a poor indicator of symptom severity, amount of reflux and oesophageal mucosal damage, and suggested that 24-hour pH is the best monitoring parameter when GER treatment is performed with the aims of improving quality of life by relieving symptoms and reversing mucosal damages.

Epidemiology of GER in Paediatrics

Patients with GER represent a major proportion of paediatric gastroenterologic practice. Older children show a disorder pattern similar to that of adults but different from that of infants. The main differences are represented by:
1. Duration: the disease tends to persist in older subjects, while in infants it generally disappears within the first two years of life [47, 48];
2. Symptoms, which in infants are mainly atypical.

To define the epidemiology in a paediatric population, patients have been categorised by specific criteria into 3 distinct groups which classify GER as functional, pathogenic or secondary [49]. Functional GER is perceived as a developmental/physiological condition mainly showing post-prandial refluxes in an otherwise well infant. This phenomenon is present in about 10%-40% of infants and its frequency significantly decreases to 4% after the sixth month of life when children start to eat solid foods [50]. Functional GER may become pathogenic during its course. Symptoms are atypical and include increasing irritability, feeding difficulty, failure to thrive, sleep disturbances, haematemesis, bronchospasm, apnoea, chronic cough (especially at night), and Sandifer's syndrome [51]. The incidence of pathogenic GER varies from 1:500 to 1:1000 [52]. In the presence of clinical signs of pathogenic GER, the possibility of concomitant oesophagitis is high [53]. Finally, secondary GER refers to the disorder affecting patients with neurological impairment. Although only 10%-15% of these patients have significant emesis [54], 70%-80% have GER as determined by pH monitoring [55].

Conclusions

Patients with GER, which include about 10%-15% of the general population, experience a considerable impairment of life quality. Effective therapy will likely result in a detectable improvement of generic measures of health status. Therefore, in an era of cost containment, the evaluation of health-related quality of life in patients with GER needs to be taken into consideration as an adequate outcome measure for the duration and the modalities of a therapy.

References

1. Kitchin LI, Castell DO (1991) Rationale and efficacy of conservative therapy for gastroesophageal reflux disease. Arch Intern Med 151:448-454
2. Vandenplas Y (1997) Oesophageal pH monitoring: how gold is the gold standard? Ital J Gastroenterol Hepatol 29:302-304
3. Vandenplas Y, Goyvaerts H, Helven R (1990) Do esophageal pH monitoring data depend on recording equipment and probes? J Pediatr Gastroenterol Nutr 10:332-336
4. Holtmann G, Goebell H, Talley NJ (1994) Dyspepsia in consulters and nonconsul-

ters. Prevalence, health care, seeking behaviour and risk factors. Eur J Gastroenterol Hepatol 6:917-924

5. Zighelboim J, Talley NJ (1993) What are functional bowel disorders? Gastroenterology 104:1196-1201

6. Talley NJ, Zinsmeister AR, Melton LJ 3rd (1995) Irritable bowel syndrome in a community: symptom subgroups, risk factors and health care utilization. Am J Epidemiol 142:76-83

7. Barlow AP, DeMeester TR, Boll CS, Eypasch EP (1989) The significance of the gastric secretory state in gastroesophageal reflux disease. Arch Surg 124:937-940

8. Katz PO, Castell DO (1998) Gastroesophageal reflux disease during pregnancy. Gastroenterol Clin North Am 27:153-167

9. McNamara DA, O'Donohoe MK, Horgan PG, et al (1998) Symptoms of oesophageal reflux are more common following laparoscopic cholecystectomy than in a control population. Ir J Med Sci 167:11-13

10. Vicari JJ, Peck RM, Falk GW, et al (1998) The seroprevalence of cagA-positive *Helicobacter pylori* strains in the spectrum of gastroesophageal reflux disease. Gastroenterology 115:50-57

11. Giannoni C, Sulek M, Friedman EM, Duncan NO (1998) Gastroesophageal reflux association with laryngomalacia: a prospective study. Int J Pediatr Otorhinolaryngol 43:11-20

12. Peters FT, Kleibeuker JH, Postma DS (1998) Gastric asthma: a pathophysiological entity? Scand J Gastroenterol 225:19-23

13. Sontag SJ (1997) Gastroesophageal reflux and asthma. Am J Med 103:84-90

14. Talley NJ, Colin-Jones D, Koch KL, et al (1991) Functional dyspepsia: a classification with guidelines for diagnosis and management. Gastroenterol Int 4:145-160

15. Locke GR, Talley NJ, Fett S, et al (1997) Prevalence and clinical spectrum of gastroesophageal reflux: a population based study in Olmsted County, Minnesota. Gastroenterology 112:1448-1456

16. Talley NJ, Boyce P, Jones M (1998) Identification of distinct upper and lower gastrointestinal symptom groupings in an urban population. Gut 42:690-695

17. Nebel OT, Frones MF, Castell DO (1976) Symptomatic gastric oesophageal reflux: incidence and precipitating factors. Dig Dis Sci 21:953-956

18. Talley NJ, Zinsmeister AR, Phillips SF, et al (1990) Prevalence of dyspepsia subgroups and their association with the irritable bowel syndrome in a community. Am J Gastroenterol 85:1241

19. Kjellen G, Tibbling L (1981) Manometric oesophageal function, acid perfusion test and symptomatology in 55 year old general population. Clin Physiol 1:405-415

20. Richter JE, Castell DO (1982) Gastroesophageal reflux. Pathogenesis, diagnosis and therapy. Ann Intern Med 97:93-103

21. Petersen H, Fjosne ULF, Johannessen T, et al (1985) Clinical significance of upper abdominal symptoms. Scand J Gastroenterol 20:19-22

22. Rex JC, Andersen HA, Bartholomew LG, Cain JC (1961) Esophageal hiatal hernia - a 10 year study of medically treated cases. J Am Med Assoc 178:117-120

23. Ollyo JB, Lang F, Fontolliet CH, et al (1990) A simple, reproducible, logical, complete and useful classification. Gastroenterology 98:A100

24. Loof L, Gotell P, Elfberg B (1993) The incidence of reflux oesophagitis. A study of endoscopy reports from a defined catchment area in Sweden. Scand J Gastroenterol 28:113-118

25. Endo M, Kobayashi S, Suzuky H, et al (1971) Diagnosis of early esophageal cancer. Endoscopy 2:61-66

26. Novis BH, Bank S, Marks IN, et al (1974) Upper gastro-intestinal fiberoptic endoscopy. S Afr Med J 48:857-861

27. Rasmussen CW (1976) A new endoscopic classification of chronic esophagitis. Am J Gastroenterol 65:409-415

28. Cronstedt J, Carling L, Vestergaard P, et al (1978) Oeophageal disease revealed by endoscopy in 1000 patients referred primarly for gastroscopy. Acta Med Scand 204:413-416

29. Tauris P (1978) Upper gastrointestinal fiberotic panendoscopy. Endoscopy 10:86-89

30. Yuguero del Moral L, Ojeda Jimenez C, Coma del Corral J, et al (1982) Esofagitis de reflujo y esofago de Barrett. Rev Esp Enf Digest 61:388-397

31. Henrion J, Heller F (1983) Endobrachy-oesophage, étude clinique et endoscopique de 22 cas. Acta Gastroenterol Belg 46:207-219

32. Aubry P, Oddes B (1984) Apport de l'endoscopie oesogastroduodenale au diagnostic en zone tropicale. Med Trop 44:231-239

33. Berstad A, Weberg R, Froyshov Larsen I, et al (1986) Relationship of hiatus hernia to reflux oesophagitis. Scand J Gastroenterol 21:55-58

34. Cooper BR, Barbezat GO (1987) Barrett's oesophagus: a clinical study of 52 patients. Q J M 62:97-108

35. Klotz F, Koutele F, L'Her P, et al (1987) La pathologie digestive haute du Gabon. Med Chir Dig 16:321-324

36. Carteret E, Pasqual JC, Renard P, et al (1988) Frequency and prognosis of erosive reflux esophagitis. Gastroenterology 94:A61

37. Kodjoh N, Hountondji A, Addra B (1991) Apport de l'endoscopie au diagnostic des affections oesogastroduodenales en milieu tropical. Ann Gastroenterol Hepatol 27:261-267

38. Baldi F, Ferrarini F, Morselli-Labate AM (1985) Prevalence of esophagitis in patients undergoing routine upper endoscopy: a multicenter survey in Italy. In: DeMeester TR, Skinner DB (eds) Esophageal disorders: pathophysiology and therapy. Raven, New York, pp 213-219

39. Ollyo JB (1986) L'oesophagite par reflux au cours du syndrome de Zollinger-Ellison. Mémoire pour le titre d'assistant étranger. Xavier Bichat, Paris, p 75

40. Stoker DL, Williams JG, Leicester RG, et al (1988) Oesophagitis: a five year review. Gut 29:A1450

41. Baldi F, Brandaccio ML (1995) Epidemiologia dell'esofagite da reflusso. In: Morelli A, Fiorucci S (eds) Malattia da reflusso gastroesofageo. EdiSES, Napoli, pp 156-158

42. Dimeneas E (1993) Methodological aspects of evaluation of quality of life in upper gastrointestinal diseases. Scand J Gastroenterol 28:18-21

43. Chal KL, Stacey JH, Sacks GE (1995) The effect of ranitidine on symptom relief and quality of life of patients with gastroesophageal reflux disease. Br J Clin Pract 49:73-77

44. Rush DR, Stelmach WJ, Young TL, et al (1995) Clinical effectiveness and quality of life with ranitidine vs placebo in gastroesophageal reflux disease patients: a clinical experience network (CEN) study. J Fam Pract 41:126-136

45. Revicki DA, Wood M, Maton PM, et al (1998) The impact of gastroesophageal reflux disease on heath-related quality of life. Am J Med 104:252-258

46. Velanovich V, Karmy-Jones R (1998) Measuring gastroesophageal disease: relationship between the health-related quality of life score and physiologic parameters. Am Surg 64:649-653

47. Carre IJ (1979) A historical review of the clinical consequences of hiatal hernia and gastroesophageal reflux. In: Gellis S (ed) Gastroesophageal reflux: Report of the 76th Ross Conference on Pediatric Research. Ross Laboratories, Columbus, pp 1-12

48. Shepherd RW, Wren J, Evans S, et al (1987) Gastroesophageal reflux in children:

clinical profile, course and outcome with active therapy in 126 cases. Clin Pediatr 26:55-60
49. Boyle JT (1989) Gastroesophageal reflux in the pediatric patient. Gastroenterol Clin North Am 18:315-337
50. Kibel MA (1979) Gastroesophageal reflux and failure to thrive in infancy. In: Gellis SS (ed) Gastroesophageal reflux: Report of the 76th Ross Conference on Pediatric Research. Ross Laboratories, Columbus, pp 39-42
51. Herbst JJ (1981) Gastroesophageal reflux. J Pediatr 98:859-870
52. Hyams JS, Ricci A Jr, Leichtner AM, et al (1988) Clinical and laboratory correlates of oesophagitis in young children. J Pediatr Gastroenterol 7:52-56
53. Shub MO, Ulshen MH, Hargrove CB (1985) Esophagitis: a frequent consequence of gastroesophageal reflux in infancy. J Pediatr 107:881-884
54. Ball TS, Hendricksen H, Clayton J (1974) A special feeding technique for chronic regurgitation. Am J Ment Defic 78:486-493
55. Sondheimer JM, Morris BA (1979) Gastroesophageal reflux among severe retarded children. J Pediatr 94:710-714

Pathophysiology of Gastroesophageal Reflux

S. Passaretti[1] and E. Strada[2]

Introduction

The gastroesophageal junction is an area of great anatomical and functional complexity whose role is to restrict physiological gastroesophageal reflux (GER) (Fig. 1). "Restricting" is the operative word inasmuch as reflux is, within certain limits, a totally physiological phenomenon. In fact, GER is assisted by the gradient between the positive pressure of the stomach (10-20 mm Hg) and the pressure of the esophagus which, as a result of intrapleural pressure, is almost always negative (ranging from 0 to -10 mm Hg). Furthermore, certain movements (e.g. inspiring, bending forward, straining, coughing) cause a marked increase in abdominal pressure. For this reason food present in the stomach would constantly rise back up into the esophagus were it not for the intervention of competence mechanisms - competence being defined as the ability to restrict and contain the incidence of gastroesophageal refluxes.

Competence mechanisms may be divided into two categories: anatomical and functional. The former comprises the angle of His, Allison's loop (serving to maintain a correct angle between the stomach and esophagus), and all the ligaments (e.g. phrenogastric, phrenoesophageal) which preserve a correct anatomical balance between the organs located in this area (Fig. 1). The latter consists essentially of the lower esophageal sphincter (LES).

The LES is 4 cm long and made up of a segment of smooth muscles. These are highly specialised and are able to maintain a state of tonic contraction which guarantees the closing of the sphincter. This is an area of high pressure, more easily identified functionally than anatomically. The phasic activity of the LES, controlled by nerves, coordinates with the act of swallowing, serving to inhibit the basal tone and to produce relaxation of the sphincter after swallowing. A variety of factors influence the basal tone of the LES, and may therefore affect, albeit indirectly, gastroesophageal reflux (Table 1).

[1]Gastroenterology Unit, Department of Science and Biomedical Technology, San Raffaele University Hospital, Milan, Italy; [2]Gastroenterology Unit, Department of Internal Medicine and Medical Oncology, Policlinico San Matteo, University of Pavia, Italy

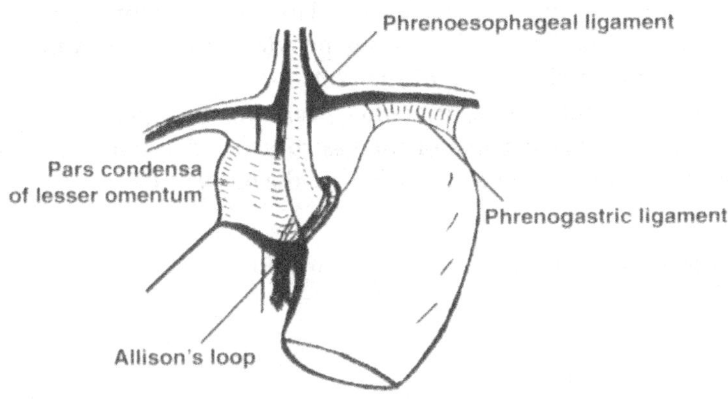

Fig. 1. Gastroesophageal junction anatomy

Table 1. Substances affecting lower esophageal sphincter pressure (LESP) and their effect on GER

	LESP	Effect on GER
Protein	↑	–
Fat	↓ ↓ ↓	–
Chocolate	↓ ↓ ↓	↑
Coffee	↑ ↓	–
Alcohol	↓ ↓ ↓	↑ ↑ ↑
Carminatives (peppermint, onion, garlic, some spices)	↓ ↓ ↓	↑ ↑ ↑
Progesterone	↓ ↓	–
Aminophyllin	↓	–
Ca^{2+} antagonists (diltiazem, nifedipine, verapamil)	↓ ↓	–
Nitroderivatives (nitroglycerin and isosorbide)	↓ ↓	–
β-adrenergics	↓	–
Dopamine	↓ ↓	–

↑ ↑ ↑, significantly increases; ↑, increases; ↑ ↓, has variable effect; ↓, decreases; ↓ ↓ ↓, significantly decreases; –, not tested

An important role in the competence of the gastroesophageal junction would appear to be played by the abdominal segment of the LES. This segment corresponds to that part of the sphincter, approximately 1-2 cm in length, located in the abdomen and thus exposed to abdominal pressure. It seems to function as a kind of flap valve which by collapsing its walls is able to adapt the pressure in the sphincter to any increases, whether gradual or sharp, in abdominal pressure. In this way it serves to guarantee successful competence of the LES.

It should also be stressed that achieving an effective antireflux barrier is greatly dependent upon the external compression exerted by the pillars of the diaphragm on the sphincter. These would appear to act as a second sphincter, helping to maintain basal pressure [1]. This fails to happen, however, in the presence of a hiatal hernia shifting the position of the LES to the point above the insertion of the diaphragm pillars [2-4].

Although the occurrence of pathological refluxes depends upon alterations in the antireflux mechanisms of the gastroesophageal junction, other factors external to the sphincter may contribute to the onset of GER (Table 2).

Table 2. Mechanisms and alterations occurring in GERD

Sphincteral

Transient relaxations of the LES
Mechanically defective sphincter
  Inadequate adaptation in the sphincter area to a rise in endogastric pressure
  ($\rightarrow$ stress reflux)
Sliding hiatus hernia
"Luxury" external factors (alcohol, smoking, mint, chocolate)
Hormonal factors
Iatrogenic factors (drugs, destruction of the LES owing to surgical resection, myotonia or pneumatic dilatation)

Extra-sphincteral

Alterations of esophageal peristalsis
Partial or total absence of salivary secretions
Delayed stomach emptying
Systemic and connectivum diseases
Pregnancy

Transient Relaxations of the LES

At present the primary cause of sphincter incompetence appears to be the so-called transient relaxations of the LES - transient and spontaneous inhibitions of the physiological sphincter tone, not associated with either swallowing nor motor waves of the esophageal body (Fig. 2) [5-11]. They lead to the formation of a clear "passage" between the stomach and esophagus, with attendant gastroesophageal reflux. They also represent a physiological response to the expanding of the base of the stomach induced by the intake of food, and are apparently responsible for the majority of occurrences of gastroesophageal reflux both in normal patients and in those with gastroesophageal reflux disease (GERD).

Mechanically Defective LES

Other frequent causes of reflux are a reduction of the basal tone or a shortening in length either of the entire sphincter or its abdominal segment, which

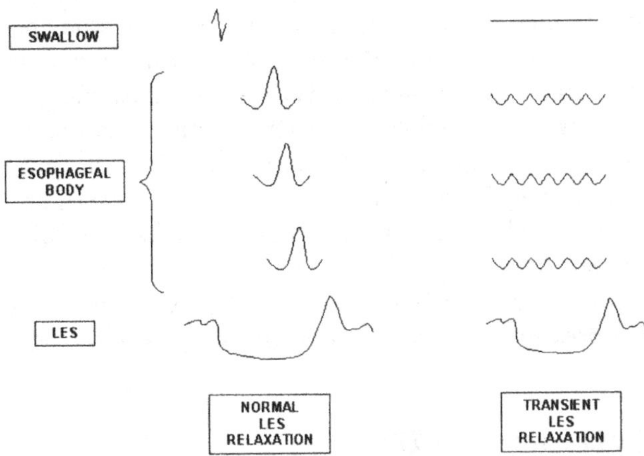

Fig. 2. Transient relaxations of LES

thus becomes mechanically defective, unable to withstand intragastric pressure or prevent the reflux of gastric material into the esophagus [3, 7, 9, 12, 13].

Reduced sphincter pressure can cause two different types of reflux: stress reflux and free reflux. The former is due to an inadequate response of the LES to a sudden rise in pressure in the abdomen (after coughing, bending etc.), while the latter is brought on by a marked sphincteral hypotony. When this happens the pressure of the LES is so low that there is no longer any barrier at all between the stomach and esophagus, which thus become a common cavity [2, 11, 12].

There is also a link between the length of the LES (and of its abdominal segment) and GER: a short sphincter or one with a short abdominal segment proves less competent and is less resistant to GER [10].

Hiatal Hernia

There exist other anatomical situations able to influence functional factors and to increase the likelihood of GER. For instance the presence of a hernia of the esophageal hiatus causes the LES to rise up into the thoracic cavity, with attendant loss of anatomical linkage between the sphincter and the pillars of the diaphragm. As mentioned earlier, the pillars play an important role in the correct functioning of the gastroesophageal junction, working in unison with the LES to create an effective antireflux barrier [14-19].

Patients with hiatal hernia, irrespective of the pressure of the LES, are subject to frequent occurrences of acidic reflux following physical effort (stress reflux) [2]. This is said to be due to the absence of the "pinchcock effect", which is created by the contraction of the diaphragm crura in physiological conditions, and which enhances the competence of the LES [13, 20].

Furthermore, hiatal hernia is said to increase the exposition time of the esophageal mucus to the refluxed material. In fact, a recent study performed on hiatal hernia patients demonstrated that during swallowing there is a re-reflux of the trapped acid from the hernia towards the esophagus, thus prolonging the period of contact between the refluxed material and the mucus [11, 21].

The above accounts for the fact that hiatal hernia is often (but not always) associated with esophagitis (with a frequency of 60%-87%), or with reflux symptoms (50%-64%), whereas in people unaffected by these phenomena its frequency is relatively low (4%-25%).

Other conditions may contribute to the onset of GER in that they cause a rise in abdominal pressure, for example pregnancy or obesity.

Extra-Sphincteral Factors and GERD

Gastroesophageal reflux is clearly the necessary and indispensable prerequisite for the occurrence of GERD. Nevertheless it is worth underlining that factors external to the sphincter may also contribute and occasionally be decisive in the onset of this disease.

The motility of the esophagus, as well as having the task of transporting the food bolus, is also responsible for clearing the esophagus of any refluxed material. This clearing activity takes place during esophageal peristalsis, which is evoked either by voluntary swallowing (primary peristalsis) or automatically when the esophageal mucus is stimulated by chemical or physical factors (secondary peristalsis). For this reason alterations in esophageal motility (anomalies in the propagation of motor waves, or propagated motor waves with low width) may hinder efficient clearing of the esophageal lumen, resulting in a longer period of contact between the damaging refluxed material and the esophageal mucus [22, 23].

Nonetheless it should not be forgotten that if the esophageal motility has the task of clearing the refluxed material, the saliva, with its alkaline pH, has the task of hindering the acidity caused by the reflux. It is therefore the case that those pathologies (in reality quite rare - for example Sjögren syndrome) or iatrogenic techniques (radiotherapy) which alter the physiological secretion of the salivary glands may be contributing factors in the development of GERD [13, 24].

The emptying of the stomach may also be an important functional factor. Gastric hypomotility or the presence of dyskinesias may hinder stomach emptying after meals, causing food in the stomach to stagnate. This in turn makes the stomach expand, triggering an increased number of inappropriate relaxations of LES. Indeed, 50% of GER patients are affected by symptoms of delayed stomach emptying (e.g. nausea, vomiting, sensation of bloating after meals) [13, 25-27]. Nevertheless, it is difficult to establish whether there is a genuine process of cause and effect in these cases, or whether the association is purely a matter of chance, given that there is a high occurrence of both types of symptoms in the population as a whole.

There is one last fundamental factor contributing to the onset of GERD: the resistance of the esophageal mucus. Unfortunately it is not possible at the present stage to measure this parameter with routine techniques.

It should be recalled that the esophageal mucous membrane is made up of a scaly, multi-layered epithelium containing rare glandular structures under the mucus able to secrete a reduced but important quantity of bicarbonates. The impermeability of the epithelium is guaranteed by tight cellular junctions, which delay the flowing back of the damaging reflux agents. Importantly, if these junctions become impaired in some way, the intercellular spaces may widen, thus rendering the mucous membrane more permeable to acid [28].

Tissue damage may be caused not only by acid but also by enzymes (pepsin and trypsin), surface-active substances (lysolecithin and bile salts), or certain characteristics of ingested materials (e.g. temperature, osmolarity).

GER pathologies can also be secondary to other pathologies affecting the physiological motility of the gastroesophageal junction or of the esophageal body, such as those involving connective tissue and smooth muscle fibres. The most important pathologies of this type are progressive systemic sclerosis (sclerodermas) and myopathies of the smooth muscles. In such cases there is a marked hypotony of the LES, as well as disturbed or absent peristalsis of the lower three-quarters of the esophageal body (made up of smooth muscle). Consequently there is a notable rise in the number of gastroesophageal refluxes owing to sphincter incompetence, plus longer duration of the refluxes themselves, as a result of alteration of the esophageal motility.

Conclusions

Until relatively recently, GERD had been principally considered a pathology resulting from the presence of hiatal hernia, from incompetence of the LES or from acidic hypersecretion. More recent physiopathological developments suggest that a variety of other factors play a part, particularly changes in functional mechanisms, which generally restrict acidic reflux.

For this reason, even though the LES still appears to be the principal cause of GER, it should be emphasised that other factors external to the sphincter, such as hernia of the esophageal hiatus or slow stomach emptying, may contribute significantly to GER. However, GER is not an automatic result of disease, which will develop only when the delicate balance between aggressive factors and defence mechanisms is upset in some way. Currently, a range of efficient endoscopic equipment is available, including the manometer, the pH metre, and the endoscope, all providing a better understanding of the mechanisms responsible for GER. Greater knowledge of these enables us to optimise and even personalise therapeutic approaches in the context of both medical and surgical therapy.

References

1. Dent J, Dodds WJ, Hogan WJ, Toouli J (1988) Factors that influence induction of gastroesophageal reflux in normal human subjects. Dig Dis Sci 33:270-275
2. Sloan S, Kahrilas PJ (1991) Hiatal hernias with or without a hypotensive LES predispose to stress reflux. Gastroenterology 100:A164
3. Sloan S, Rademaker AW, Kahrilas PJ (1992) Determinants of gastroesophageal junction incompetence. Hiatal hernia, lower esophageal sphincter or both? Ann Intern Med 117:977-982
4. Sloan S, Kahrilas PJ (1991) Impairment of esophageal emptying with hiatal hernia. Gastroenterology 100:596-605
5. Mittal RK, Holloway RH, Penagini R, Blackshaw LA, Dent J (1995) Transient lower esophageal sphincter relaxation. Gastroenterology 109:601-610
6. Dent J, Dodds WJ, Friedman RH, Sekiguchi T, Hogan WJ, Arndorfer RC, Petrie DJ (1980) Mechanism of GER in recumbent asymptomatic human subjects. J Clin Invest 65:256-267
7. Dodds WJ, Dent J, Hogan WJ, Helm JF, Hauser R, Patel GK, Egide MS (1982) Mechanisms of gastroesophageal reflux in patients with reflux esophagitis. N Engl J Med 307:1547-1552
8 Dodds WJ, Kahrilas PJ, Dent J, Hogan WJ, Kern MK, Arndorfer RC (1989) Analysis of spontaneous gastroesophageal reflux and esophageal acid clearance in patients with reflux esophagitis. J Gastrointest Motil 2:79-81
9. Dent J, Holloway RH, Toouli J, Dodds WJ (1988) Mechanisms of lower oesophageal sphincter incompetence in patients with symptomatic gastroesophageal reflux. Gut 29:1020-1028
10. Mittal RK, McCallum RW (1987) Characteristics of transient lower esophageal sphincter relaxation in humans. Am J Physiol 252:g636-g641
11. Schaub N (1985) Pathogenesis of gastroesophageal reflux. Schweiz Med Wochenschr 115:114-125
12. Kahrilas PJ (1997) Anatomy and physiology of the gastroesophageal junction. Gastroenterol Clin North Am 26:467-486
13. Galmiche JP, Janssens J (1995) The pathophysiology of gastro-oesophageal reflux disease: an overview. Scand J Gastroenterol Suppl 211:7-18
14. DeMeester TR, Lafontaine E, Joelsson BE, et al (1981) Relationship of a hiatal hernia to the function of the body of the esophagus and the gastroesophageal junction. J Thorac Cardiovasc Surg 82:547-558
15. Cohen S, Harris LD (1971) Does hiatus hernia affect competence of the gastroesophageal sphincter? N Engl J Med 284:1053-1056
16. Santos GH (1983) Is hiatus hernia responsible for reflux? Chest 84:242-244
17. Ellis FH (1972) Esophageal hiatal hernia. N Engl J Med 287:646-649
18. Kaul B, Petersen H, Myrovold HE, Grette K, Roysland P, Halvorsen T (1986) Hiatus hernia in gastroesophageal reflux disease. Scand J Gastroenterol 21:31-34
19. Berstad A, Webweg R, Froyshov Larsen I, Hoel B, Hauer-Jensen M (1986) Relationship of hiatus hernia to reflux esophagitis. A prospective study of coincidence using endoscopy. Scand J Gastroenterol 21:55-58
20. Mittal RK (1990) Current concepts of the antireflux barrier. Gastroenterol Clin North Am 19:501-516
21. Mittal RK, Lange RC, McCallum RW (1987) Identification and mechanism of delayed gastric esophageal clearance in subjects with hiatus hernia. Gastroenterology 92:130-135

22. Kahrilas PJ, Dodds WJ, Hogan WJ, Kern M, Arndorfer RC, Reece A (1996) Esophageal peristaltic dysfunction in peptic esophagitis. Gastroenterology 91:897-904

23. Olsen AM, Schlegel JF (1965) Motility disturbances caused by esophagitis. J Thorac Cardiovasc Surg 50:607-612

24. Helm JF, Dodds WS, Pelc LR, et al (1984) Effect of esophageal emptying and saliva on clearance of acid from the esophagus. N Engl J Med 310:284-288

25. Sontag SJ (1993) Rolling review: gastro-oesophageal reflux disease. Aliment Pharmacol Ther 7:293-312

26. McCallum RW, Berkowitiz DM, Lerner E (1981) Gastric emptying in patients with GER. Gastroenterology 80:285-291

27. Cunningham KM, Horowitz M, Riddell PS, Maddern GJ, Myers JC, Holloway RH, Wishart JM, Jamieson GG (1991) Relations among autonomic nerve dysfunction, oesophageal motility, and gastric emptying in gastro-oesophageal reflux disease. Gut 32:1436-1440

28. Tobey NA, Carson JL, Alkiek RA, Orlando RC (1996) Dilated intercellular spaces: a morphological feature of acid reflux--damaged human esophageal epithelium. Gastroenterology 111:1200-1205

Gastroesophageal Reflux in Pneumology

Pathophysiological Determinants of Gastroesophageal Reflux, and the Role of Esophageal and Airway Receptors

G. Sant'Ambrogio and F.B. Sant'Ambrogio

Introduction

Although the human body is well equipped to counteract the occurrence of a reflux of gastric contents into the esophagus and possibly into the more proximal airway, regurgitation does occur, especially in elderly subjects and in newborns. In healthy subjects, physiological mechanisms offer a well-developed degree of protection against gastroesophageal reflux (GER) as shown by its absence even in subjects maintained in a head-down posture [1]. The most common disorder leading to GER is a functional or structural abnormality of the lower esophageal sphincter affecting either one of its two components: smooth muscle or striated muscle from the crural portion of the diaphragm [1].

It has been known for a long time that several impairments of the respiratory tract (i.e. bronchoconstriction, laryngospasm) are associated with GER [2-5]. However, it is still a matter of debate whether these disorders depend on reflexes originating from esophageal or airway receptors [6-8]; it has indeed been proven that the gastric refluxate can reach different portions of the proximal airway [9].

In view of the possibility that some of the responses to GER originate through the stimulation of esophageal receptors, one should (a) consider the properties of esophageal afferent endings and (b) compare the responses to acidic solutions instilled into the esophagus to those obtained with laryngeal instillation. Another possible consequence of GER is the harmful effect that acidic solutions might have on some laryngeal reflex functions such as those related to the maintenance of upper airway patency.

Department of Physiology and Biophysics, University of Texas Medical Branch, Galveston, Texas, USA

Properties of Esophageal Receptors of Dogs: Mechanical and Chemical Responsiveness

The vagal afferent innervation of the esophagus seems to be relatively scant when compared to other portions of the alimentary tract [10]. Esophageal vagal receptors with myelinated fibers have been characterized in several animal species [11-15]. Most of the esophageal receptors are localized in the intrathoracic portion of the esophagus and respond to a maintained distension of the esophageal wall with the characteristic behavior of slowly adapting afferent endings (SAR) [14-16]. Since esophageal distension, the most effective way to activate them, leads to reflex responses of upper airway and respiratory muscles that resemble those of deglutition [17], we may reasonably presume that these endings are involved in the mechanism of swallowing [12]. Far less numerous are the rapidly adapting endings (RAR) that exhibit an "on" and "off" response to esophageal distension [16].

Sekizawa et al. [15] found that of 24 SARs and 4 RARs challenged with a solution of hydrochloric acid and pepsin (pH = 1), only 2 SARs and 1 RAR were specifically stimulated; the same receptors were also challenged with distilled water and none was activated. Of 5 SARs and 2 RARs exposed to topically applied capsaicin, only 1 RAR was stimulated.

In conclusion, the esophagus seems to have scant vagal innervation with a preponderance of SARs possibly involved in the mechanisms of deglutition. Especially relevant to our interest is the poor response of esophageal receptors to acidic solutions and other irritants. Altogether, these results do not support an important reflexogenic role of the esophagus in response to chemical irritants.

Larynx and Esophagus as Reflexogenic Sites for Acid-Induced Bronchoconstriction in Dogs

Bronchoconstriction is frequently associated with GER in asthmatic patients [3, 9, 18, 19]. It is still controversial whether this reflex originates from the esophagus or from aspiration of the refluxate into the larynx and lower airway [6-8]. As a matter of fact, the larynx is an important reflexogenic site and acid-induced laryngitis is frequently observed in GER patients [20, 21].

Ishikawa et al. [22], in order to address this point, compared the effects of repeated esophageal and laryngeal instillations of HCl-pepsin (to mimic gastric juice) on tracheal smooth muscle activity in anesthetized and artificially ventilated dogs. Cuff pressure of an endotracheal tube (Pcuff) was used as an index of smooth muscle activity [23]. Esophageal instillations of either HCl-pepsin or saline, used as control, did not change Pcuff (Fig. 1). HCl-pepsin instilled into the larynx elicited a prompt and sustained contraction of the trachealis muscle; repeated administrations enhanced the responsiveness significantly. Saline instillations elicited only small and transient responses probably due to mechanical stimulation (Fig. 1).

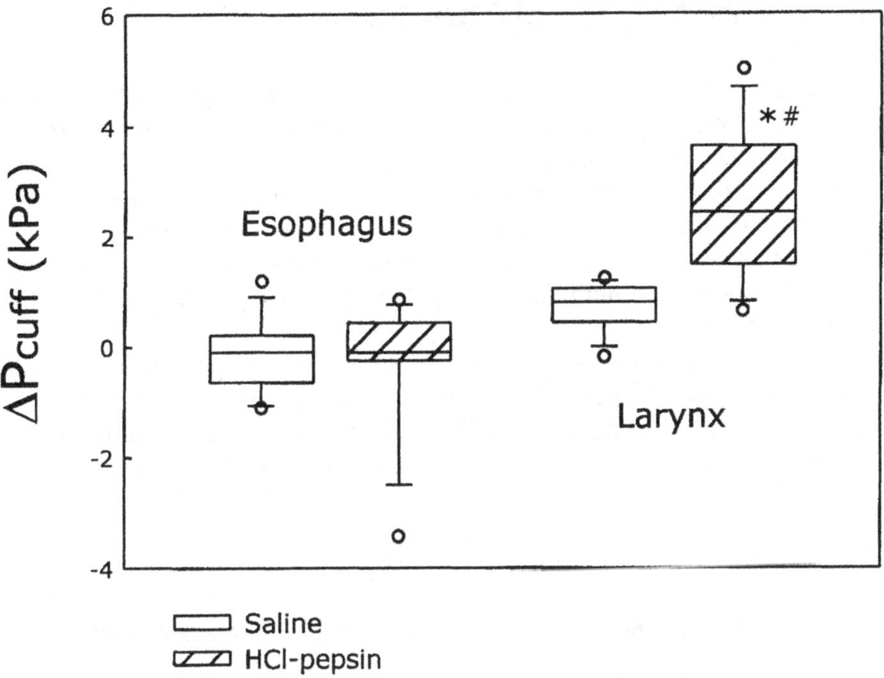

Fig. 1. Box plot representing the effect of esophageal and laryngeal HCl-pepsin instillations on tracheal smooth muscle activity. *∆Pcuff*, change from the baseline pressure of the cuff of an endotracheal tube placed in the extrathoracic trachea. Pcuff is used as an indication of smooth muscle activity. The horizontal lines on each box represent, from bottom to top, 25th, 50th and 75th percentiles. Bars represent the 10th and 90th percentiles, and circles the lowest and highest values. *, significant difference between the effect of esophageal and laryngeal HCl-pepsin instillations; #, significant difference between saline and HCl-pepsin laryngeal instillations

It is therefore clear that, at least in the dog, the esophagus can hardly qualify as a reflexogenic site for the elicitation of reflex bronchoconstriction in response to acidic solutions. This is in agreement with the findings by Tuchman et al. [7] who reported that the increase in total lung resistance was three-times higher with tracheal infusion than with esophageal infusion. Bilateral section of the vagus nerves eliminated the response. Similar indications can be derived from a study by Tatár and Pécová [24] who found that intraesophageal instillations of hydrochloric acid did not induced cough in anesthetized cats. Indeed, the number and nature of the esophageal receptors found and characterized in previous studies [14-16] could have anticipated the results of the reflex studies.

Impairment of Patency-Maintaining Mechanisms

The larynx is endowed with different types of afferent endings; slowly adapting mechanoreceptors responsive to negative pressure are particularly well represented among laryngeal endings [25].

The posterior cricoarytenoid muscle (PCA) and other upper airway abductors increase their activity when the upper airway is subjected to negative pressure [26-29]. The activity of laryngeal mechanoreceptors is well related to that of the PCA. The same stimuli that modify their discharge also modify the activity of the PCA [25].

The gastroesophageal refluxate can involve upper airway structures and damage the laryngeal mucosa [5, 30]. It seems reasonable to propose that the function of laryngeal receptors and thus that of patency-maintaining mechanisms might also be compromised. This was demonstrated in a canine experi-

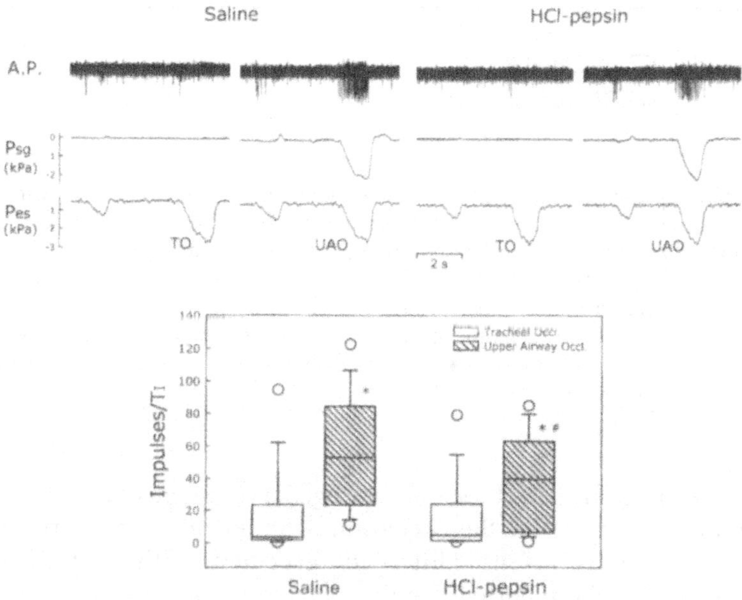

Fig. 2. Effect of repeated laryngeal instillations of HCl-pepsin (pH = 2) on negative pressure-responsive receptors. *Upper panel,* experimental record showing action potentials (*A.P.*), subglottic pressure (*Psg*) and esophageal pressure (*Pes*). *Lower panel,* box plot summarizing the data on afferent endings. See Fig. 1 for details on this type of representation. The response of the afferent endings to laryngeal negative pressure is measured by the difference between the activity during tracheal occlusion (*TO,* no changes in pressure across the larynx) and upper airway occlusion (*UAO,* larynx exposed to collapsing pressure). Laryngeal instillations of HCl-pepsin (2 or 3 trials) severely impair the response of laryngeal afferent endings to negative pressure. *, statistically significant difference between tracheal and laryngeal occlusion; #, statistically significant difference between saline and HCl-pepsin instillations

mental model [31]. The larynx, exposed to repeated instillations of solutions similar in composition to gastric juice (HCl-pepsin), sustained extensive inflammatory and necrotic alterations at the level of the mucosa. After 2-3 instillations, the response of laryngeal receptors to negative pressure decreased to 68% (Fig. 2). When the activity of the PCA was assessed, it was found that after four instillations its response to upper airway occlusion, a maneuver that exposes the larynx to negative pressure, was severely compromised. In fact, there was no longer a statistical difference with the discharge of the PCA in response to tracheal occlusion, a maneuver that elicits the same inspiratory efforts, but does not change the pressure across the larynx. Successive instillations further decreased the response to negative pressure (Fig. 3).

Since the activity of the upper airway patency-maintaining muscle decreases during sleep [26] and GER occurs more frequently during the night [18], one can see how this damage to the upper airway patency-maintaining mechanism can escalate. Elderly, obese, asthmatic people, persons prone to sleep apnea, and pregnant women are particularly at risk [18, 32-34].

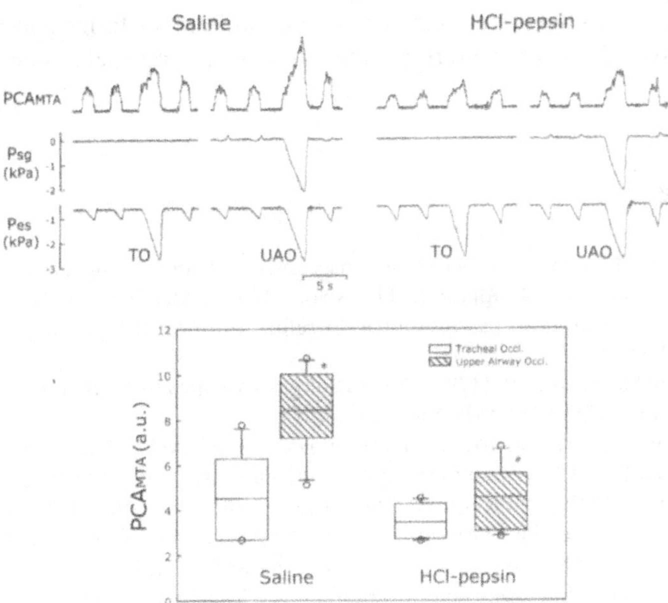

Fig. 3. Effect of repeated laryngeal instillations of HCl-pepsin (pH = 2) on PCA activity. *Upper panel*, experimental record showing the moving time average of the posterior cricoarytenoid muscle electromyograms (*PCAmta*), subglottic pressure (*Psg*) and esophageal pressure (*Pes*). *TO*, tracheal occlusion; *UAO*, upper airway occlusion. *Lower panel*, box plot summarizing the data of these experiments; see Fig. 1 for details. The 6th instillation of HCl-pepsin abolishes the PCA response to upper airway occlusion (no difference between tracheal and upper airway occlusion). *, statistically significant difference between tracheal and laryngeal occlusion; #, statistically significant difference between saline and HCl-pepsin instillations

Conclusions

Results obtained in animal models indicate that gastric content regurgitation limited to the esophagus does not induce bronchoconstriction. On the other hand, when it reaches the larynx it does elicit bronchoconstriction, and the response increases with repeated exposures. As compared to the esophagus, the larynx appears to be a clearly reactive site. This is in accordance with the much greater number of laryngeal than esophageal rapidly adapting (irritant) receptors. After all, it would seem inappropriate for the esophagus to be too reactive to substances (e.g. water, acidic solutions) that are present in food that it is normally swallowed as a bolus.

Regurgitation of gastric juice may affect the larynx in a way that is detrimental to its reflex functions. The experimental results considered herein prove the presence of mucosal damage even after limited exposure to HCl-pepsin solutions. GER should be viewed as a condition that can either initiate or aggravate the occurrence of upper airway obstruction.

One could also envisage the possibility that other reflex functions, besides the laryngeal patency-maintaining mechanism, be affected by GER. For instance, if the cough reflex is impaired (due to damage to irritant receptors), the refluxate might reach more peripheral airways and make more extensive damage.

References

1.   Mittal RK, Balaban DH (1997) The esophagogastric junction. N Engl J Med 336:924-932
2.   Boyle JT, Tuchman DN, Altschuler SM, Nixon TE, Pack AI, Cohen S (1985) Mechanisms for the association of gastroesophageal reflux and bronchospasm. Am Rev Respir Dis 131:S16-S20
3.   Harding SM, Richter JE (1997) The role of gastroesophageal reflux in chronic cough and asthma. Chest 111:1389-1402
4.   Kahrilas PJ (1996) Gastroesophageal reflux disease. JAMA 276:983-988
5.   Koufman JA (1991) The otolaryngologic manifestations of gastroesophageal reflux disease (GERD): a clinical investigation of 255 patients using ambulatory 24-hour pH monitoring and an experimental investigation of the role of acid and pepsin in the development of laryngeal injury. Laryngoscope 101:1-78
6.   Schan CA, Harding SM, Haile JM, Bradley LA, Richter JE (1994) Gastroesophageal reflux-induced bronchoconstriction. An intraesophageal acid infusion study using state-of-the-art technology. Chest 106:731-737
7.   Tuchman DN, Boyle JT, Pack AI, Scwartz J, Kokonos M, Spitzer AR, Cohen S (1984) Comparison of airway responses following tracheal or esophageal acidification in the cat. Gastroenterology 87:872-881
8.   Wesseling G, Brummer RJ, Wouters EF, ten Velde GP (1993) Gastric asthma? No change in respiratory impedance during intraesophageal acidification in adult asthmatics. Chest 104:1733-1736
9.   Donnelly RJ, Berrisford RG, Jack CI, Tran JA, Evans CC (1993) Simultaneous tracheal and esophageal pH monitoring: investigating reflux-associated asthma. Ann

Thorac Surg 56:1029-1034

10. Paintal AS (1963) Vagal afferent fibres. In: Kramer K, Krayer O, Lehnartz E, Muralt A, Weber HH (eds) Ergebnisse der Physiologie, Band 52. Springer, Berlin Heidelberg New York, pp 74-156

11. Andrews PL, Lang KM (1982) Vagal afferent discharge from mechanoreceptors in the lower oesophagus of the ferret. J Physiol (Lond) 322:29P

12. Clerc N, Mei N (1983) Vagal mechanoreceptors located in the lower oesophageal sphincter of the cat. J Physiol (Lond) 336:487-498

13. Falempin M, Mei N, Rousseau JP (1978) Vagal mechanoreceptors of the inferior thoracic oesophagus, the lower oesophageal sphincter and the stomach in the sheep. Pflügers Arch 373:25-30

14. Satchell PM (1984) Canine oesophageal mechanoreceptors. J Physiol (Lond) 346: 287-300

15. Sekizawa S-I, Ishikawa T, Sant'Ambrogio FB, Sant'Ambrogio G (1998) Vagal esophageal receptors in the anesthetized dog. FASEB J 12:A782

16. Mei N (1970) Mécanorécepteurs vagaux digestifs chez le chat. Exp Brain Res 11: 502-514

17. Cherniack NS, Haxhiu MA, Mitra J, Strohl K, Van Lunteren E (1984) Responses of upper airway, intercostal and the diaphragm muscle activity to stimulation of oesophageal afferents. J Physiol (Lond) 349:15-25

18. Ayres JG, Miles JF (1996) Oesophageal reflux and asthma. Eur Respir J 9:1073-1078

19. Mays EE (1976) Intrinsic asthma in adults. Association with gastroesophageal reflux. JAMA 236:2626-2628

20. Olson NR (1991) Laryngopharyngeal manifestations of gastroesophageal reflux disease. Otolaryngol Clin North Am 24:1201-1213

21. Sataloff RT, Speigel JR, Hawkshaw M, Rosen DC (1993) Gastroesophageal reflux laryngitis. Ear Nose Throat J 72:113-114

22. Ishikawa T, Sekizawa S-I, Sant'Ambrogio FB, Sant'Ambrogio G (1998) Effect of esophageal vs. laryngeal HCl-pepsin instillations on airway smooth muscle in adult dogs. FASEB J 12:A784

23. Ishikawa T, Sekizawa S, Sant'Ambrogio FB, Sant'Ambrogio G (1998) Endotracheal cuff pressure as an index of airway smooth muscle activity: comparison with total lung resistance. Respir Physiol 112:175-184

24. Tatár M, Pécová R (1996) The effect of experimental gastroesophageal reflux on the cough in anesthetized cats. Bratisl Lek Listy 5:284-288

25. Sant'Ambrogio G, Tsubone H, Sant'Ambrogio FB (1995) Sensory information from the upper airway: role in the control of breathing. Respir Physiol 102:1-16

26. Kuna ST, Sant'Ambrogio G (1991) Pathophysiology of upper airway closure during sleep. JAMA 266:1384-1389

27. Mathew OP, Abu-Osba YK, Thach BT (1982) Influence of upper airway pressure changes on genioglossus muscle respiratory activity. J Appl Physiol 52:438-444

28. Sant'Ambrogio FB, Mathew OP, Clark WD, Sant'Ambrogio G (1985) Laryngeal influences on breathing pattern and posterior cricoarytenoid muscle activity. J Appl Physiol 58:1298-1304

29. Van Lunteren E, Van de Graaff WB, Parker DM, Mitra J, Haxhiu MA, Strohl KP, Cherniack NS (1984) Nasal and laryngeal reflex responses to negative upper airway pressure. J Appl Physiol 56:746-752

30. Chodosh PL (1977) Gastro-esophago-pharyngeal reflux. Laryngoscope 87:1418-1427

31. Sant'Ambrogio FB, Sant'Ambrogio G, Chung K (1998) Effects of HCl-pepsin laryngeal instillations on upper airway patency-maintaining mechanisms. J Appl Physiol 84:1299-1304

32. Feinberg MJ, Knebl J, Tully J, Segall L (1990) Aspiration in the elderly. Dysphagia 5:61-71
33. Hagen J, Deitel M, Khanna RK, Ilves R (1987) Gastroesophageal reflux in the massively obese. Int Surg 72:1-3
34. Nebel OT, Fornes MS, Castell DO (1976) Symptomatic gastroesophageal reflux: incidence and precipitating factors. Am J Dig Dis 21:953-956

The Role of Protons in the Activation of Primary Sensory Neurons

P. Geppetti, S. Amadesi, M. Tognetto, and F.M.L. Ricciardolo

Capsaicin-Sensitive Primary Sensory Neurons

Primary sensory neurons with cell bodies localized to trigeminal, vagal and dorsal root ganglia (DRG) consist of different subpopulations of pseudounipolar neurons distinguished according to their phenotype, velocity of impulse conduction, neurotransmitter content and type of stimulus that they recognize. Among these diverse subpopulations, a group of neurons exists that are uniquely stimulated by capsaicin and that express and release from their central and peripheral terminals neuropeptide transmitters. Capsaicin, better known as the hot principle contained in the plants of the genus *Capsicum*, is a vanilloid derivative that exerts multiple and specific actions on primary sensory neurons [1]. These actions somehow resemble those exerted by guanethidine on sympathetic neurons. At low concentrations, capsaicin excites neurons of in vitro preparations by promoting cation influx (Na^+ and Ca^{2+}) into the nerve terminal. This event initiates a propagated action potential that orthodromically invades the neurons, thus conveying the sensory information to the lamina I and II of the dorsal spinal cord and medulla oblongata. The consequence of this effect (often appreciated when small quantities of capsaicin are added to food) is a hot and burning sensation that usually fades in a few minutes without any appreciable tissue damage.

However, the propagated action potential may also antidromically invade collateral fibers of the arborized terminal region of the neurons, thus depolarizing these collateral fibers. Ca^{2+} influx, both caused by the direct action of capsaicin at its site of stimulatory action and consequent to the opening of voltage-sensitive Ca^{2+} channels due to the depolarizing stimulus, promotes two different effects. First, it triggers the release of peptide transmitters from nerve fiber varicosities at the peripheral and central levels. Second, when high concentrations of capsaicin are used, the massive influx of Ca^{2+} (a concentration as high

Department of Experimental and Clinical Medicine, Pharmacology Unit, University of Ferrara, Italy

as 12 mM intracellular Ca^{2+} has been measured upon neuronal stimulation with
$> \mu M$ capsaicin) [2] into the cell induces a series of events including osmotic
changes and protease activation that cause cell death. The possibility to selectively stimulate and/or kill a specific subset of neurons has made capsaicin a
unique tool for studying the physiologic functions and the pathophysiologic
involvement of this subpopulation of primary sensory neurons and their neuropeptide transmitters.

The ability of high doses of capsaicin (if administered to newborn rats) to
permanently destroy a subpopulation of primary sensory neurons, sensitive to
its excitotoxic action, has given the opportunity to define precisely their characteristics [1]. Capsaicin-sensitive primary sensory neurons belong to a subpopulation of neurons with small and dark cell bodies and with unmyelinated or
thinly myelinated fibers of the $A\delta$ and C types that contain neuropeptides.
These neurons are activated by diverse nociceptive stimuli, namely heat, high
threshold mechanical stimuli and chemical stimuli. Therefore, they have been
referred to as polymodal nociceptors. These properties have been defined mainly
in small rodents. However, capsaicin-sensitive and neuropeptide-containing primary sensory neurons have been found in all mammals, including man. The
widespread use of creams or ointments containing capsaicin for treating various painful and non-painful human diseases derives from the old observation
of the popular medicine that continuous administration of small doses of certain algesic substances may reduce pain (counterirritation). However, progress
in understanding the molecular mechanism of capsaicin action has suggested
that its beneficial effect in certain diseases, including post-herpetic neuralgia or
post-mastectomy pain, may rely on its ability to specifically desensitize the sub-
population of neurons that it excites [3]. It is possible that the small doses of
topical capsaicin used for treatment of human disease are not able (as observed
in adult rats) to kill sensory neurons, but rather they cause a more subtle type
of desensitization [4, 5]. However, no convincing molecular mechanism that can
clarify the therapeutic action of capsaicin has been proposed yet.

Neurogenic Inflammation

A number of neuropeptides are expressed by primary sensory neurons [6].
However, for only a few have Ca^{2+}-dependent release and physiologic functions
been demonstrated. These neuropeptides include calcitonin gene-related peptide (CGRP) and the tachykinins substance P (SP) and neurokinin A (NKA).
CGRP is the product of the alternative splicing of the calcitonin gene, an event
that occurs selectively in the nervous system [7]. The 38 amino acid peptide
CGRP is also present in intrinsic neurons of the gut and in neurons of the central nervous system. CGRP activates different receptors which were first characterized on a pharmacological basis as the $CGRP_1$ and $CGRP_2$ receptors. The

recent discovery that intracellular regulatory proteins called RAMP [8] may modify the unique molecular entity representing the CGRP/amylin receptor into various conformers that bind with different affinities the various endogenous agonists has spread new light on the unresolved issue of CGRP receptor subtypes. CGRP is the most powerful vasodilator known [9]. It causes positive inotropic and chronotropic effects in the heart, relaxes or contracts certain non-vascular smooth muscles (urinary bladder and iris, respectively) [10, 11], and exerts some metabolic effects [12].

The other neuropeptides released from central and peripheral endings of primary sensory neurons are SP and NKA. These peptides belong to a large family of small peptides, called tachykinins, that share a common C-terminus sequence and that are present in a large variety of species from amphibians to mammals [13]. Another important member of this family is neurokinin B (NKB). However, because its precursor, produced by the pre-pro-tachykinin B gene, is not expressed in peripheral neurons it does not have any apparent role in the peripheral nervous system. Tachykinins stimulate three types of receptors, namely the NK_1, NK_2 and NK_3 receptors [14]. NK_1 receptors are activated by all the three tachykinins with similar potency [15], whereas NK_2 and NK_3 receptors are preferentially activated by NKA and NKB, respectively. SP and NKA released from terminals of primary sensory neurons in peripheral tissues causes all the major signs of inflammation via the activation of NK_1 and NK_2 receptors. These signs include plasma protein extravasation in post-capillary venules (NK_1), arteriolar vasodilatation (NK_1), leukocyte adhesion to the endothelium of post-capillary venules (NK_1) and activation of inflammatory cells ($NK1_1$). Tachykinins may also cause tissue-specific effects. For instance, in the airways they cause contraction (mainly NK_2, but also NK_1) or relaxation (NK_1) of tracheobronchial smooth muscle cells, secretion from seromucous cells (NK_1), hyperresponsiveness following a variety of stimuli (NK_2 and NK_1), and cough (mainly NK_2, but also NK_1) [16].

A number of mediators and agents have been found to stimulate neuropeptide release from peripheral terminals of primary sensory neurons, thus causing a series of inflammatory responses collectively referred to as "neurogenic inflammation" [6, 17]. Many of the stimuli found to stimulate neurogenic inflammatory responses in the airways of experimental animals are also of pathophysiological relevance in human airway diseases. For instance, plasma protein extravasation caused by inhalation of cigarette smoke in rodents was completely blocked by capsaicin pretreatment [18] or by a selective NK_1 receptor antagonist [19]. A large part of the bronchoconstriction and plasma extravasation caused by exposure of sensitized guinea pigs to antigen challenge is due to activation of NK_2 and NK_1 receptors, respectively [20, 21]. Finally, the increase in bronchoconstriction and plasma extravasation that follows inhalation of cold air, a stimulus that can worsen attacks of asthma, was abolished by NK_2 and NK_1 receptor antagonists, respectively [22, 23].

Protons as Stimulants of Primary Sensory Neurons

A huge number of stimuli has been found to stimulate primary sensory neurons and to cause neurogenic inflammatory responses [6, 24]. Low pH medium is included in this long list, as increasing proton concentrations can activate primary sensory neurons to release sensory neuropeptides [25]. The pH of plasma is adjusted rapidly by renal and respiratory mechanisms. Hence, it is unlikely that the small variations in plasma pH that occur systemically may stimulate primary sensory neurons. However, in certain conditions, either physiological or pathological, the pH of the medium may be low enough to stimulate primary sensory neurons and cause the release of proinflammatory neuropeptides. The first indirect evidence of this phenomenon was obtained in rats: the inflammatory response in the rat peritoneum after injection of acetic acid [26], and the plasma extravasation caused by instillation of acidic solution into the trachea [27] were abolished by capsaicin pretreatment (Fig. 1). The first direct evidence of the ability of protons to cause transmitter secretion from sensory neu-

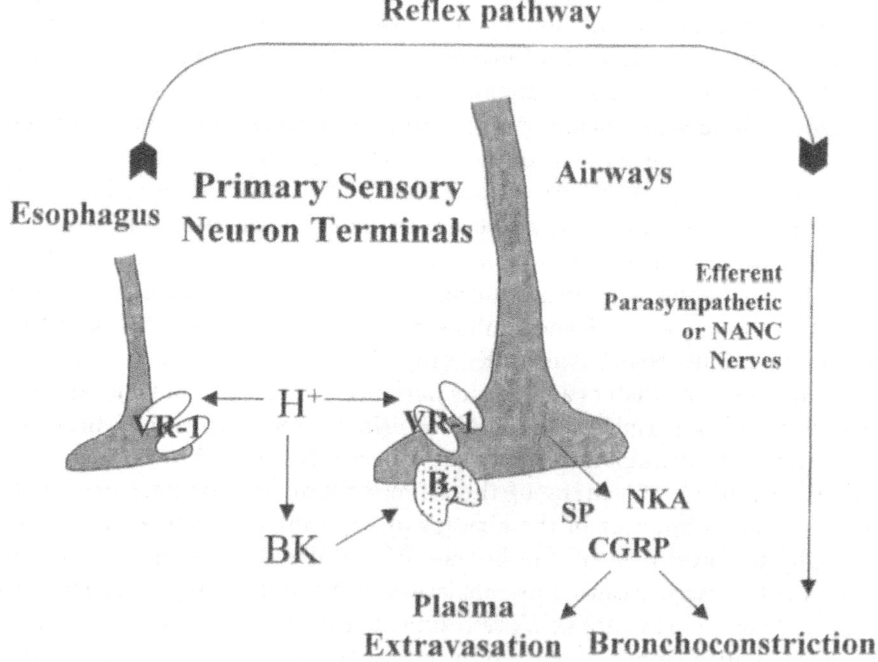

Fig. 1. Proposed mechanisms by which acidic media cause bronchoconstriction and inflammation in the airways. Increased proton (H^+) concentrations in the airways (caused by aspiration of acid material into the trachea) cause, by direct stimulation of the vanilloid receptor/channel (*VR-1*) or via bradykinin (*BK*) formation, the release of tachykinins (*SP* and *NKA*) and CGRP and the subsequent bronchoconstriction and inflammation. Alternatively, bronchoconstriction may be caused by the presence of acidic fluid in the lower esophagus and is mediated by a reflex pathway. *NANC*, nonadrenergic noncholinergic

rons was obtained from slices of guinea-pig urinary bladder: exposure of this tissue to media at pH 6 or 5 caused a pH-dependent increase in CGRP outflow. The observation that CGRP release caused by low pH was abolished in a Ca^{2+}-free medium and after capsaicin pretreatment indicated that protons do not damage the tissue, but rather activate a neurosecretory Ca^{2+}-dependent process [28, 29]. The ability of protons to release CGRP or SP has been also demonstrated in other tissues of rat and guinea pig. These include the stomach [30], heart [31], airways [32], skeletal muscle [33], dural venous sinuses [34] and dorsal spinal cord [35].

An important question is that relative to the selectivity of proton action on primary sensory neurons as protons may also stimulate other neurons in the central and peripheral nervous systems. In the rat stomach, a large quantity of CGRP is contained in terminals of capsaicin-sensitive primary sensory neurons, whereas the bulk of SP is present in capsaicin-insensitive intrinsic neurons of the stomach [30]. Media at pH 6 or 5 were able to stimulate the release of CGRP, but not of SP, from slices of rat stomach [30]. This observation favors the hypothesis that protons exhibit a certain degree of selectivity in releasing peptides, and their action is mainly directed to those neurons that are stimulated by capsaicin.

The Molecular Basis of Capsaicin and Proton Action on Primary Sensory Neurons

In a large number of afferent neurons, step changes in pH (to pH 7.0) induce transient currents that inactivate within 5 s. These currents result from the activation of a channel selectively permeable to Na^+. A second type of current is detected in a smaller population of neurons that seems to coincide with the capsaicin-sensitive population. This sustained current is a result of the activation of ion channels that are permeable to Na^+, K^+ and Ca^{2+}, and is only elicited by large changes in pH (to < pH 6.5) that are not required to be rapid [36]. The profile of this current makes it a good candidate to explain the sustained afferent discharge seen in rat skin-nerve preparations and the sustained pain response observed after injection of low pH solution (pH 5.2) into the human skin [37]. The molecular mechanisms that underlie the excitation of primary sensory neurons by protons have not been clarified, although some information has been provided by recent studies.

Ruthenium red, in a narrow range of concentrations, selectively antagonized the $^{45}Ca^{2+}$ uptake induced by capsaicin in DRGs by interfering with ion channel activity [2]. Capsazepine, a structural analogue of capsaicin, acts as a selective antagonist of capsaicin [38, 39]. There is evidence showing that ruthenium red and capsazepine antagonize responses elicited by protons. In rodents, ruthenium red and capsazepine rather selectively inhibited contraction of bronchial smooth muscle, CGRP release from skeletal muscle, various smooth muscle responses, and nasal irritation induced by either capsaicin or protons [28, 40-42]. This evidence suggests that protons and capsaicin activate a common mechanism that is sensitive to ruthenium red and capsazepine. Electrophysiological studies confirmed this view only partially: while low capsazepine concentrations inhibited proton-induced currents in trigeminal neurons [43], proton-induced activation of a rat tail-spinal cord preparation and ion influx in cultured DRG neurons were not blocked by capsazepine (A. Dray and H.P. Rand, unpublished observations).

Recently, the rat gene coding the capsaicin-activated receptor/channel has been cloned [44]. This channel, denominated vanilloid receptor-1 (VR-1), belongs to the family of store-activated channels and is permeable to cations. Studies performed in Xenopus oocytes transfected with VR-1 indicated that this channel has all the characteristics of the capsaicin-activated channel in DRGs, including sensitivity to ruthenium red and capsazepine. The channel was stimulated by heat, but not by protons alone. However, protons sensitized the channel to stimulation by other agents including heat. It is tempting to speculate that protons sensitize DRG discharge even at physiological temperatures (37° C) that normally maintain quiescent neuronal activity. Finally, the possibility that molecular entities sensitive to capsaicin other than VR-1 exist makes the situation more complex than originally thought.

Pathophysiological Significance of Proton Action on Primary Sensory Neurons: Gastroesophageal Reflux in Asthma

Sensory neurons may be exposed to low pH media in pathological conditions. Thus, acidic conditions have been implicated in the inflammatory exudates of synovial fluid in arthritis [45], and in the venous effluent from ischemic areas [46]. Increased proton concentrations occur not only in pathological states but also under normal physiological conditions in the stomach and urinary bladder lumen and in skeletal muscle during anaerobic work. Following damage to the gastric or bladder mucosa, protons (pH 2-5) may diffuse into the tissue in concentrations sufficient to stimulate the terminals of primary afferents. In the stomach, this stimulation represents a defense mechanism. In fact, proton-induced release of CGRP causes hyperemia of the stomach mucosa, an effect that has been considered protective against further tissue damage and ulcer formation [47]. Diffusion of low pH urine to the sensory nerve terminal after urothelium damage can be associated with discomfort, pain and cystitis.

A strong association has been reported between gastroesophageal reflux (GER) and asthma [48, 49]. Although patients in antireflux therapy do not have demonstrable changes in lung function, their asthma symptoms improve [48, 49]. Although it is not clear which mechanism is responsible for the association between GER and asthma, two main hypotheses have been proposed. The first suggests that tracheal aspiration of gastric contents may stimulate a local inflammatory reaction. The second proposes that the presence of acid in the lower esophagus triggers a vagally mediated bronchospasm. Although the second of these two hypotheses can not presently be rejected, much evidence has been accumulated in experimental animal models to favor the first hypothesis.

There is convincing data that a direct action of protons on sensory nerves is responsible for the neurogenically mediated inflammatory response in airways. For instance, local instillation of acid into the trachea of rats or guinea pigs increases plasma protein extravasation [27] and bronchoconstriction [42], both effects being blocked by tachykinin receptor antagonists and by capsazepine [42]. However, there is also proof that in certain experimental conditions, possibly dependent upon the actual proton concentration in the milieu other mechanisms may be activated. In a recent study, bronchoconstriction induced by an aerosol of citric acid was abolished by a tachykinin B_2 receptor antagonist and was inhibited by a bradykinin B_2 receptor antagonist [50]. This finding argues against the proposal that the sole mechanism of acid-induced bronchoconstriction is a direct role of protons on sensory nerve terminals. It is possible that kinins formed after exposure to acid stimulate, via B_2 receptor activation, NKA and SP release that increases bronchial smooth muscle tone.

Conclusions

In an elegant experiment, Fischer et al. showed that guinea pig neurons intrinsic to the esophagus and containing NO and vasoactive intestinal polypepeptide project axons to the adjacent trachealis where they produce relaxation [51]. From these studies it is tempting to speculate that excitatory nerves may also directly project from the esophagus to the tracheobronchial wall. These fibers might be involved in acid-induced bronchoconstriction. Alternatively, either a reflex pathway connecting esophageal afferents or parasympathetic or nonadrenergic-noncholinergic efferent nerve fibers in the airways may be involved. Finally, the direct presence of acid in the tracheobronchial lumen may stimulate sensory nerve terminals in the mucosa. However in man none of these mechanisms has been conclusively demonstrated. Therefore, more studies are required to clarify whether a direct (inspiration of acid into the airways) or indirect mechanism is involved in GER-induced asthma attacks. More studies are also required to determine which kind of neural connection exists between the gastroesophageal and airway tissues. However, the studies summarized in the present chapter underline the primary role of acidic media in triggering inflammatory responses via a neurogenic mechanism. These studies also point to the possibility that acid-induced and neurogenic-mediated inflammation has a role in the worsening of asthma associated with GER.

Acknowledgements. This paper was supported by grants from CNR, Rome, Italy and by Azienda Ospedaliera Sant'Anna, Ferrara, Italy.

References

1. Holzer P (1991) Capsaicin: cellular targets, mechanisms of actions, and selectivity for thin sensory neurons. Pharmacol Rev 43:143-201
2. Wood JN, Winter J, James IF, Rang HP, Yeats J, Bevan S (1988) Capsaicin-induced ion fluxes in dorsal root ganglion cells in culture. J Neurosci 8:3208-3220
3. Geppetti P (1996) Capsaicin as a drug. In: Geppetti P, Holzer P (eds) Neurogenic inflammation. CRC, Boca Raton, pp 289-298
4. Dray A, Bettaney J, Forster P (1989) Capsaicin desensitization of peripheral nociceptive fibres does not impair sensitivity to other noxious stimuli. Neurosci Lett 99: 50-54
5. Dray A (1992) Mechanism of action of capsaicin-like molecules on sensory neurons. Life Sci 51:1759-1765
6. Holzer P (1988) Local effector functions of capsaicin-sensitive sensory nerves endings: involvement of tachykinins, calcitonin gene-related peptide and other neuropeptides. Neuroscience 24:739-768
7. Amara SG, Jonas V, Rosenfeld MG, Ong ES, Evans RM (1982) Alternative RNA processing in calcitonin gene expression generates mRNAs encoding different polypeptide products. Nature 298:240-244
8. McLatchie LM, Fraser NJ, Main MJ, Wise A, Brown J, Thompson N, Solari R, Lee MG, Foord SM (1998) RAMPs regulate the transport and ligand specificity of the calcitonin-receptor-like receptor. Nature 393:333-339
9. Brain SD, Williams TJ, Tippins JR, Morris HR, MacIntyre I (1985) Calcitonin gene-related peptide is a potent vasodilator. Nature 313:54-56
10. Maggi C, Giuliani S (1991) The neurotransmitter role of calcitonin gene-related peptide in the rat and guinea-pig ureter: effect of calcitonin gene-related peptide antagonist and species-related differences in the action of omega conotoxin on calcitonin gene-related peptide release from primary afferents. Neuroscience 43:261-268
11. Geppetti P, Patacchini R, Cecconi R, Tramontana M, Meini S, Romani A, Nardi M, Maggi CA (1990) Effects of capsaicin, tachykinins, calcitonin gene-related peptide and bradykinin in the pig iris sphincter muscle. Naunyn Schmiedebergs Arch Pharmacol 341:301-307
12. Hall JM, Brain SD (1996) Pharmacology of calcitonin gene-related peptide. In: Geppetti P, Holzer P (eds) Neurogenic inflammation. CRC, Boca Raton, pp 101-114
13. Otsuka M, Yoshioka K (1993) Neurotransmitter functions of mammalian tachykinins. Physiol Rev 73:229-308
14. Regoli D, Boudon A, Fauchere J-L (1994) Receptors and antagonists for substance P and related peptides. Pharmacol Rev 46:551-599
15. Maggi CA, Schwartz TW (1997) The dual nature of the tachykinin NK_1 receptor. Trends Pharmacol Sci 18:351-355
16. Advenier C, Daoui S, Cui YY, Lagente V, Emonds-Alt X (1996) Inhibition by the tachykinin NK_3 receptor antagonist, SR 142801, of substance P-induced microvascular leakage hypersensitivity and airway hyperresponsiveness in guinea-pigs. Am J Respir Crit Care Med 153:A163
17. Szolcsanyi J (1984) Capsaicin-sensitive chemoceptive neural system with dual sensory-efferent function. In: Chahl LA, Szolcsanyi J, Lembeck F (ed) Antidromic vasodilatation and neurogenic inflammation. Akademiai Kiado, Budapest, pp 27-56
18. Lundberg JM, Saria A (1983) Capsaicin induced desensitization of the airway mucosa to cigarette smoke, mechanical and chemical irritants. Nature 302:251-253
19. Delay-Goyet P, Lundberg JM (1991) Cigarette smoke-induced airway oedema is blocked by the NK1 antagonist, CP-96,345. Eur J Pharmacol 203:157-158

20. Bertrand C, Geppetti P, Graf PD, Nadel JA (1993) Involvement of neurogenic inflammation in antigen-induced bronchoconstriction in guinea pigs. Am J Physiol 265:L507-L511

21. Kudlacz EM, Knippenberg RW, Logan DE, Burkholder TP (1996) Effect of MDL 105,212, a nonpeptide NK-1/NK-2 receptor antagonist in an allergic guinea pig model. J Pharmacol Exp Ther 279:732-739

22. Yoshihara S, Chan B, Yamawaki I, Geppetti P, Riccardolo FLM, Massion P, Nadel JA (1995) Plasma extravasation in the rat trachea induced by cold air is mediated by tachykinin release from sensory nerves. Am J Respir Crit Care Med 151:1011-1017

23. Yoshihara S, Geppetti P, Hara M, Linden A, Ricciardolo FL, Chan B, Nadel JA (1996) Cold air-induced bronchoconstriction is mediated by tachykinin and kinin release in guinea pigs. Eur J Pharmacol 296:291-296

24. Maggi C (1991) The pharmacology of the efferent function of sensory nerves. J Auton Pharmacol 11:173-208

25. Bevan S, Geppetti P (1994) Protons, small stimulants of capsaicin-sensitive sensory nerves. Trends Neurosci 17:509-512

26. Arvier PT, Chahl LA, Ladd RJ (1977) Modification by capsaicin and compound 48/80 of dye leakage induced by irritants in the rat. Br J Pharmacol 59:61-68

27. Martling C-R, Lundberg JM (1988) Capsaicin sensitive afferents contribute to acute airway edema following tracheal instillation of hydrochloric acid or gastric juice in the rat. Anesthesiology 68:350-356

28. Geppetti P, Del Bianco E, Patacchini R, Santicioli P, Maggi CA, Tramontana M (1991) Low pH-induced release of calcitonin gene-related peptide from capsaicin-sensitive sensory nerves: mechanism of action and biological response. Neuroscience 41:295-301

29. Geppetti P, Tramontana M, Patacchini R, Del Bianco E, Santicioli P, Maggi CA (1990) Neurochemical evidence for the activation of the 'efferent' function of capsaicin-sensitive nerves by lowering of the pH in the guinea-pig urinary bladder. Neurosci Lett 114:101-106

30. Geppetti P, Tramontana M, Evangelista S, Renzi D, Maggi CA, Fusco BM, Del Bianco E (1991) Differential effect on neuropeptide release of different concentrations of hydrogen ions on afferent and intrinsic neurons of the rat stomach. Gastroenterology 101:1505-1511

31. Franco-Cereceda A, Lundberg JM (1992) Capsazepine inhibits low pH- and lactic acid-evoked release of calcitonin gene-related peptide from sensory nerves in guinea-pig heart. Eur J Pharmacol 221:183-184

32. Lou YP, Lundberg JM (1992) Inhibition of low pH evoked activation of airway sensory nerves by capsazepine, a novel capsaicin-receptor antagonist Biochem Biophys Res Commun 189:537-544

33. Santicioli P, Del Bianco E, Geppetti P, Maggi CA (1992) Release of calcitonin gene-related peptide-like immunoreactivity (CGRP-LI) from rat isolated soleus muscle by low pH, capsaicin and potassium. Neurosci Lett 143:19-22

34. Fanciullacci M, Tramontana M, Del Bianco E, Alessandri M, Geppetti P (1991) Low pH medium induces calcium dependent release of CGRP from sensory nerves of guinea-pig dural venous sinuses. Life Sci 49:PL27-30

35. Del Bianco E, Santicioli P, Tramontana M, Maggi CA, Cecconi R, Geppetti P (1991) Different pathways by which extracellular Ca^{2+} promotes calcitonin gene-related peptide release from central terminals of capsaicin-sensitive afferents of guinea-pigs: effect of capsaicin high K^+ and low pH media. Brain Res 566:46-53

36. Bevan S, Yeats J (1991) Protons activate a cation conductance in a sub-population of

rat dorsal root ganglion neurones. J Physiol (Lond) 433:145-161

37. Steen KH, Reeh PW (1993) Sustained graded pain and hyperalgesia from harmless experimental tissue acidosis in human skin. Neurosci Lett 154:113-116

38. Bevan S, Hothi S, Hughes G, James IF, Rang HP, Shah K, Walpole CS, Yeats JC (1992) Capsazepine: a competitive antagonist of the sensory neurone excitant capsaicin. Br J Pharmacol 107:544-552

39. Walpole CS, Bevan S, Bovermann G, Boelsterli JJ, Breckenridge R, Davies JW, Hughes GA, James I, Oberer L, Winter J, et al (1994) The discovery of capsazepine, the first competitive antagonist of the sensory neuron excitants capsaicin and resiniferatoxin. J Med Chem 37:1942-1954

40. Santicioli P, Del Bianco E, Figini M, Bevan S, Maggi CA (1993) Effect of capsazepine on the release of calcitonin gene-related peptide-like immunoreactivity (CGRP-LI) induced by low pH, capsaicin and potassium in rat soleus muscle. Br J Pharmacol 110:609-612

41. Belvisi MG, Miura M, Stretton D, Barnes PJ (1992) Capsazepine as a selective antagonist of capsaicin-induced activation of C-fibres in guinea-pig bronchi. Eur J Pharmacol 215:341-344

42. Satoh H, Lou Y-P, Lundberg JM (1993) Inhibitory effects of capsazepine and SR 48968 on citric acid-induced bronchoconstriction in guinea-pigs. Eur J Pharmacol 236:367-372

43. Liu L, Simon SA (1994) A rapid capsaicin-activated current in rat trigeminal ganglion neurons. Proc Natl Acad Sci U S A 91:738-741

44. Caterina MJ, Schumacher MA, Tominaga M, Rosen TA, Levine JD, Julius D (1997) The capsaicin receptor: a heat-activated ion channel in the pain pathway. Nature 389:816-824

45. Stevens CR, Williams RB, Farrell AJ, Blake DR (1991) Hypoxia and inflammatory synovitis: observations and speculation. Ann Rheum Dis 50:124-132

46. Jacobus WE, Taylor GJT, Hollis DP, Nunnally RL (1977) Phosphorus nuclear magnetic resonance of perfused working rat hearts. Nature 265:756-758

47. Holzer P (1998) Neural emergency system in the stomach. Gastroenterology 114:823-839

48. Sontag SJ (1997) Gastroesophageal reflux and asthma. Am J Med 103:84S-90S

49. Simpson WG (1995) Gastroesophageal reflux disease and asthma: diagnosis and management. Arch Intern Med 155:798-804

50. Ricciardolo FLM, Rado V, Fabbri LM, Sterk PJ, Di Maria GU, Geppetti P (1999) Bronchoconstriction induced by citric acid inhalation in guinea pigs. Role of tachykinins, bradykinin and nitric oxide. Am J Respir Crit Care Med 159:557-562

51. Fischer A, Canning BJ, Undem BJ, Kummer W (1998) Evidence for an esophageal origin of VIP-IR and NO synthase-IR nerves innervating the guinea pig trachealis: a retrograde neuronal tracing and immunohistochemical analysis. J Comp Neurol 394:326-334

An Ovine Model of GERD-Induced Bronchoconstriction

M. Scuri[1], L. Allegra[1], R.W. Dal Negro[2], C. Pomari[2], and W.M. Abraham[3]

Introduction

The association between bronchial asthma and gastroesophageal reflux disease (GERD) has been reported repeatedly over the last 30 years [1-6], although the issue of cause and effect remains controversial. Reports about a certain kind of relationship between asthma and GERD date back to 1912 when Sir William Osler [7] stated that "asthma attacks may be due to direct irritation of the bronchial mucosa or ... indirectly, too, by reflex influences from the stomach". Dr. Osler's insight about acid-induced bronchoconstriction remains true today. GERD, the retrograde movement of gastric contents into the esophagus, is a prevalent clinical condition affecting millions of adults around the world. An epidemiologic study performed in the USA in the 1970s suggested that 10% of the population has daily heartburn and more than one-third have intermittent symptoms [8]. More recently, another survey reported that 20% of 800 randomly selected adults had heartburn more than three times a month and another 25% noted heartburn at least once a month [9]. Untreated GERD impairs quality of life and can lead to esophageal complications such as esophagitis, ulceration, stricture and Barrett's esophagus (replacement of squamous epithelium with columnar epithelium) with its tendency to become malignant [10]. However, the spectrum of problems associated with GERD has expanded to extraesophageal sites [11]. Chronic cough and asthma are two clinical problems caused or triggered by GERD [12, 13]. Furthermore, treatment of GERD may result in marked improvement or even disappearance of symptoms in patients with chronic cough or asthma [12, 14]. One potentially critical consideration is that many asthmatic patients do not have classic reflux symptoms but only occasional asymptomatic regurgitation. This condition, although being able to

[1]Institute of Respiratory Diseases, University of Milan, IRCCS Ospedale Maggiore, Milan, Italy; [2]Lung Department, Bussolengo General Hospital, Bussolengo (Verona), Italy; [3]University of Miami at Mount Sinai Medical Center, Miami Beach, Florida, USA

elicit cough and asthma, leaves the clinician unaware that GERD may be playing a crucial role in their patients' symptoms [15, 16].

Three potential mechanisms have been hypothesized to explain acid-induced bronchoconstriction in asthmatics. These mechanisms include: (1) a vagally mediated reflex, (2) heightened bronchial reactivity and (3) microaspiration of gastric acid resulting in bronchoconstriction [17]. Many studies show the importance of a vagally mediated reflex in GERD-induced bronchoconstriction since the esophagus and the bronchial tree share embryonic origins and autonomic innervation. Mansfield and Stein showed, in a dog model, an increase in respiratory resistance after acid infusion in the esophagus [5]. This response was ablated by bilateral vagotomy. Mansfield et al. showed similar findings in subsequent human studies [18]. In another study by Wright et al. [19] on 136 subjects, airflow and arterial oxygen saturation were significantly reduced after esophageal acid infusion. Atropine pretreatment abolished these findings, providing more evidence for an acid-induced vagally mediated esophagobronchial reflex. Although there is increasing evidence to confirm the importance of this reflex mechanism in acid-induced bronchoconstriction, other authors failed to demonstrate a significant change in airflow and/or pulmonary resistance after acid infusion of the esophagus [20].

The second hypothesized mechanism is increased bronchial hyperresponsiveness (BHR). Pomari et al. [21] found an enhanced response to methacholine in GERD patients while Herve et al. [22] showed that esophageal acid stimulation aggravates asthma by increasing bronchomotor responsiveness to other stimuli. The proposed mechanism is the interaction of esophageal acid-sensitive receptors with cholinergic bronchial tone by a vagally mediated reflex.

The third mechanism is microaspiration. "Aerosolized" acid that forms in the stomach can be aspirated into the trachea in the presence of an incontinent lower esophageal sphincter (LES). Trachea acidification is a potent bronchoconstrictive stimuli as demonstrated by Chernow et al. [23], Tuchman et al. [24], and Jack et al. [25] in both human and animal models. Furthermore, according to Tuchman et al., the esophageal acid response occurred in 60% of the animals vs. 100% of the animals with tracheal acid. Allegra et al. (unpublished data) detected radioactive coloid in lung scans of patients with GERD 24 h after instillation of the radionuclide in the stomach. In summary, esophageal acid has proved to cause bronchoconstriction probably via a vagally mediated response; however, if microaspiration is present, there is further augmentation of this bronchoconstrictor response [17].

Despite all the evidence about GERD-induced asthma, there are still controversies about the role played by acid reflux in asthmatic bronchoconstriction. In fact, it has also been suggested that it is not reflux that causes asthma but rather asthma that predisposes to increased gastroesophageal reflux. Physiological alterations associated with asthma and bronchodilator medications may in fact promote GERD [17]. In the literature one can find evidence supporting the role of asthma medications or increased transdiaphragmatic pressure as a predisposing factor for GERD [26-29]. Other authors, however, found no significant changes in the number or duration of the reflux episodes after treatment with antiasthmatic drugs [30, 31]. The issue is therefore rather complicated and controversial. A suitable experimental model would then be of great use in investigating the mechanisms responsible for this pathologic condition.

Humans pose the obvious limit of ethicity and complacency of the subject to undergo invasive procedures such as esophageal and tracheal pH monitoring, or acidification of esophagus and trachea. Animal models have been extensively used to study GERD-induced bronchoconstriction [24, 32-34]. They have provided precious information about GERD-induced asthma but have limitations varying from species to species, most notably the impossibility to study the animal while awake and, in many cases, the need to open the chest for measuring pulmonary flow resistance. As far as we know, the sheep has never been used as an experimental model for such studies. The sheep is already known as an experimental model for studying bronchial asthma [35]. Besides being capable of developing an asthmatic response to antigen challenge (*Ascaris suum*) that has many similarities with the antigen-induced bronchoconstriction in humans, it also offers the possibility of measuring pulmonary mechanics while the animal is awake. We, then, became attracted to the idea of studying the mechanisms of GERD-induced bronchospasm in this animal to evaluate its suitability for these experiments. The following is a brief description of the findings we made using the sheep as an animal model for GERD-induced bronchoconstriction.

Materials and Methods

Six adult sheep weighing 23.5-49.0 kg (mean, 32.7 kg) and with previously documented airway hypersensitivity to inhaled *Ascaris suum* antigen were used. The sheep were conscious during the study.

Measurement of Airway Mechanics

Each sheep was restrained on a cart in an upright position with its head immobilized. After topical anesthesia of the nasal passages with 2% lidocaine solution, a balloon catheter was advanced through the right nostril into the lower esophagus. The animals were intubated with a cuffed endotracheal tube through the other nostril, using a flexible fiberoptic bronchoscope. Pleural pressure was measured via an esophageal balloon catheter filled with 1 ml air, which was positioned 5-10 cm from the gastroesophageal junction. Lateral pressure in the trachea was measured with a sidehole catheter (inner dimension, 2.5 mm) advanced through and positioned distally to the tip of the endotracheal tube (Fig. 1). Transpulmonary pressure, the difference between tracheal and pleural pressure, was measured with a differential pressure transducer catheter system that showed no phase shift between pressure and flow to a frequency of 9 Hz. For measurement of the pulmonary resistance (R_L), the proximal end of the

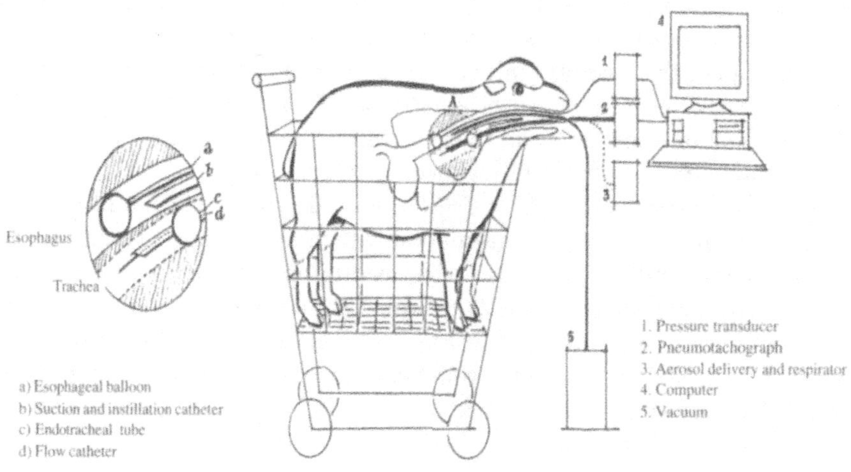

Fig. 1. System used to assess pulmonary mechanics, deliver aerosols and instill acid solutions into the esophagus of the sheep

endotracheal tube was connected to a pneumotachograph (Fleisch; Dyna Sciences, Blue Bell, PA). The signals of flow and transpulmonary pressure were recorded on an oscilloscope recorder, which was linked to a computer for online calculation of R_L. Respiratory volume was obtained by digital integration of the flow signal and was used, together with transpulmonary pressure and flow, to derive R_L. For measurement of specific lung resistance (SR_L), thoracic gas volume (Vtg) was measured in a constant-volume body plethysmograph, immediately after determining R_L.

Aerosol Delivery Systems

All aerosols were generated using a disposable medical nebulizer (Raindrop, Puritan Bennett, Lenexa, KS). The output of the nebulizer was directed into a plastic T-piece, which interconnected the inspiratory port of a Harvard respirator (Harvard Apparatus, South Natick, MA) with the animal's tracheal tube. To control aerosol delivery, a dosimeter system consisting of a solenoid valve and a source of compressed air (20 psi) was used. The solenoid valve was activated for 1 s at the beginning of the inspiratory cycle of the respirator. Aerosols were delivered at a tidal volume of 500 ml and a rate of 20 breaths/min.

Airway Responsiveness

To assess airway responsiveness, we performed cumulative dose-response curves to carbachol by measuring SR_L immediately after inhalation of buffer and after each consecutive administration of 10 breaths of increasing concentrations of carbachol up to 4% wt/vol [36]. The provocation test was discontinued when SR_L increased more than 400% from the post-saline value, or after the highest carbachol concentration had been administered. Airway responsiveness was estimated by determining the cumulative carbachol dose (in breath units), which increased SR_L by 400% over the post-saline value (PC_{400}), by interpolation from the dose-response curve. One breath unit (BU) was defined as one breath of an aerosol solution containing 1% wt/vol carbachol.

Esophagus Acid Instillation

The instillation of acid into the esophagus was performed via a catheter advanced through the right nostril and positioned about 5 cm above the balloon catheter (Fig. 1). This catheter is already used to measure mechanics and is connected with a vacuum to make the esophageal walls collapse around the balloon catheter and to avoid sheep from swallowing. The catheter was used for instillation when not measuring pulmonary mechanics.

Protocol

Acid solutions at pH 7, 5, 3.5 and 2, and 1 N HCl were given orally and by inhalation in different days. R_L was measured in baseline conditions and after every treatment. Bronchial hyperresponsiveness (assessed by cumulative carbachol dose-response curve) was measured in baseline condition and 24 h after acid inhalation. All solutions were prepared with glacial HCl diluted with saline and adjusted for pH.

Results

The ingestion or inhalation of acid solutions at pH 7, 5, or 3.5 produced little or no change at all of R_L. The instillation of acid at pH 2 and of 1 N HCl into the esophagus by means of the second esophageal catheter caused a mean increase in R_L by 117% and 182%, respectively ($p < 0.001$ vs. baseline) (Fig. 2). The aerosolization of the same solutions (30 breaths) caused a mean R_L increase of 120% and 201%, respectively ($p < 0.001$ vs. baseline) (Fig. 3). Bronchial hyperresponsiveness (BHR) measured by cumulative carbachol dose-response curve and performed 24 h after inhalation of the acid solutions was significantly higher compared to a baseline test ($p < 0.02$ vs. baseline) (Fig. 4).

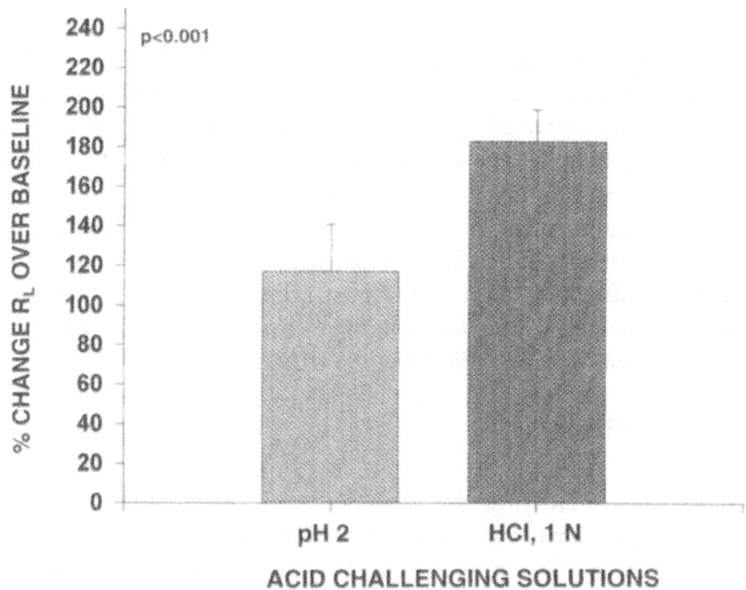

Fig. 2. The effect of acid instillation into the esophagus on pulmonary resistance (R_L). Data are expressed as % change over baseline and are mean +/- SE for six sheep. The results of two different acid solutions are shown: pH 2 and 1 N HCl

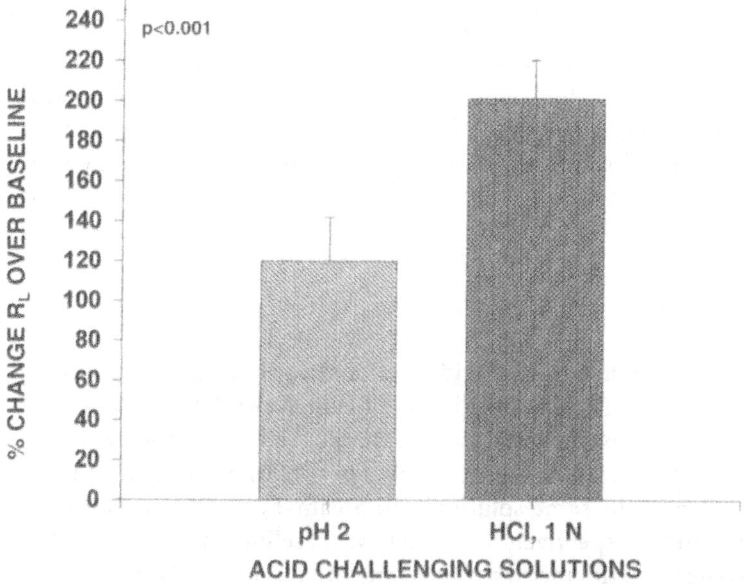

Fig. 3. The effect of tracheal acidification on pulmonary resistance (R_L). Data are expressed as % change over baseline and are mean +/- SE for six sheep. Acid solutions were delivered by aerosol. The results of two different acid solutions are shown: pH 2 and 1 N HCl

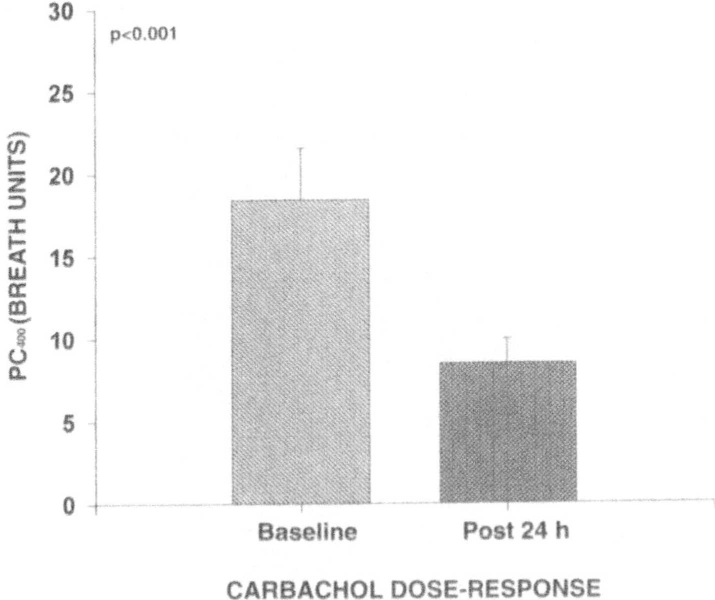

Fig. 4. Carbachol dose-response as measured in baseline conditions and 24 h after tracheal acidification. PC_{400} is the concentration of carbachol, expressed in breath units, required to increase pulmonary resistance (R_L) by 400%. One breath unit (BU) is defined as one breath of an aerosol solution containing 1% wt/vol carbachol

Discussion

The first consideration that can be made in light of the results of this study is that we were able to elicit a measurable, yet short-lived bronchospasm after challenging the esophagus and the airway with acid. This is consistent with the results of many human studies in which esophageal and tracheal acidification resulted in increased total pulmonary resistance [18]. A second important observation is that tracheal acidification produces a higher degree of bronchoconstriction than does esophageal acid instillation (182% vs. 201% when giving 1 N HCl) (Fig. 5). These data seem to confirm previous observations [24] and may provide evidence to support the microaspiration theory as one of the mechanisms involved in GERD-induced bronchoconstriction. In our ovine model we also demonstrated a heightened bronchial reactivity 24 h after challenging the airways with acid solutions. These results appear to be matching those of Herve et al. [22] and Pomari et al. [21] obtained in asthmatic subjects with acid reflux. The increase in BHR after tracheal acidification appears, in our opinion, a potentially crucial finding. Along with the indirect evidence of microaspiration, it can provide evidence for a chronic exposure of the airway mucosa to irritating factors (HCl, gastric enzymes and other potentially irritat-

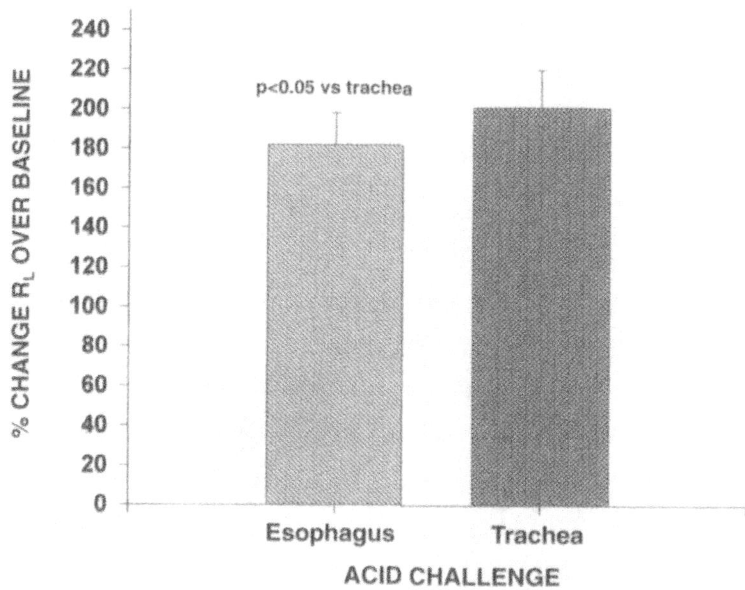

Fig. 5. Comparison of the effects of instillation into the esophagus and aerosolization of 1 N HCl on pulmonary mechanics. Data are expressed as % change of pulmonary resistance over baseline and are mean +/- SE

ing factors from the stomach) which, in turn, cause and sustain inflammation of the airways. The bronchial hyperresponsiveness, thus, can be responsible for the persistence of pulmonary symptoms even in absence of acid reflux. Although the sheep cannot be compared to humans or other mammals such as cats and dogs in terms of anatomy and physiology of the gastrointestinal tract, the responses of the airways to esophageal and tracheal acid instillation are consistent with those of other experimental models, most notably humans. Furthermore, as already noted, the sheep offers the great advantage of assessing pulmonary mechanics while the animal is awake, avoiding the potential interference of anesthetic drugs with the response of the animal to different stimuli. Also, the size of the animal offers practical advantages in terms of setting up devices for measuring pulmonary mechanics, if compared to other small animals such as cats, dogs or rats. The anatomy and physiology of the respiratory system of the sheep is fairly comparable to that of humans and, more importantly, the bronchial response to antigen challenge is qualitatively overlapping that of asthmatic patients. In conclusion, this study offers interesting, yet preliminary data indicating microaspiration and BHR as crucial factors in GERD-induced asthma. Furthermore, it indicates that the sheep is a reasonable and reliable experimental model for studying the mechanisms responsible for acid-induced bronchoconstriction. Further investigations must be done to elucidate the nature of this affection and to confirm the results of the literature.

References

1. Kennedy JH (1962) Silent gastroesophageal reflux: an important but little known cause of pulmonary complications. Dis Chest 42:42-45
2. Overholt RH, Voorhees RJ (1966) Esophageal reflux as a trigger in asthma. Dis Chest 49:464-466
3. Mays EE (1976) Intrinsic asthma in adults: association with gastroesophageal reflux. JAMA 236:2626-2628
4. Urschel HC, Paulson DL (1967) Gastroesophageal reflux and hiatal hernia: complications and therapy. J Thorac Cardiovasc Surg 53:21-32
5. Mansfield LE, Stein MR (1978) Gastroesophageal reflux and asthma: a possible reflex mechanism. Ann Allergy 41:224-726
6. Barish CF, Wu WC, Castell DO (1985) Respiratory complications of gastroesophageal reflux. Arch Intern Med 145:1882-1888
7. Osler WB (1912) The principles and practice of medicine, 8th edn. Appleton, New York, pp 628-631
8. Nebel OT, Fornes MF, Castell DO (1976) Symptomatic gastroesophageal reflux. Incidence and precipitating factors. Dig Dis Sci 21:953-956
9. A Gallup survey on heartburn across America (1988) The Gallup Organization, Princeton NJ
10. Richter JE, Castell DO (1982) Gastroesophageal reflux: pathogenesis, diagnosis and therapy. Ann Intern Med 97:93-103
11. Deschner WK, Benjamin SB (1989) Extraesophageal manifestations of gastroesophageal reflux disease. Am J Gastroenterol 84:1-5
12. Irwin RS, French CL, Curley FJ, et al (1993) Chronic cough due to gastroesophageal reflux: clinical, diagnostic, and pathogenetic aspects. Chest 104:1511-1517
13. Harding SM, Richter JE (1992) Gastroesophageal reflux disease and asthma. Semin Gastrointest Dis 3:139-150
14. Harding SM, Richter JE, Guzzo MR (1996) Asthma and gastroesophageal reflux: acid suppressive therapy improves asthma outcome. Am J Med 100:395-405
15. Irwin RS, Zawacki JK, Curley FJ, et al (1989) Chronic cough as the sole presenting manifestation of gastroesophageal reflux. Am Rev Respir Dis 140:1294-1300
16. Irwin RS, Curley FJ, French CL (1993) Difficult-to-control asthma: contributing factors and outcome of a systematic management protocol. Chest 103:1662-1669
17. Harding SM, Richter JE (1997) The role of gastroesophageal reflux in chronic cough and asthma. Chest 111:1389-1402
18. Mansfield LE, Hameister HH, Spaulding MS, et al (1981) The role of the vagus nerve in airway narrowing caused by intraesophageal hydrochloric acid provocation and esophageal distention. Ann Allergy 47:431-434
19. Wright RA, Miller SA, Corsello BF (1990) Acid-induced esophagobronchial cardiac reflexes in humans. Gastroenterology 99:71-73
20. Tan WC, Martin RJ, Pandy R, et al (1990) Effects of spontaneous and stimulated gastroesophageal reflux on sleeping asthmatics. Am Rev Respir Dis 141:1394-1399
21. Pomari GC, Micheletto C, Turco P, Dal Negro RW, et al (1995) Acid drink enhances methacholine responses in GER only in subjects showing hypoxic response to ultrasonically nebulized distilled water. Eur Respir J 10(25):66s
22. Herve P, Denjean A, Jian R, et al (1986) Intraesophageal perfusion of acid increases the bronchomotor response to methacholine and to isocapnic hyperventilation in asthmatic subjects. Am Rev Respir Dis 134:986-989
23. Chernow B, Johnson LF, Janowitz WR, et al (1979) Pulmonary aspiration as a conse-

quence of gastroesophageal reflux: a diagnostic approach. Dig Dis Sci 24:839-844

24. Tuchman DN, Boyle JT, Pack AL, et al (1984) Comparison of airways responses following tracheal or esophageal acidification in the cat. Gastroenterology 87:872-881

25. Jack CIA, Calverley PMA, Donnelly RJ, et al (1995) Simultaneaous tracheal and esophageal pH measurements in asthmatic patients with gastroesophageal reflux. Thorax 50:201-204

26. Zfass AM, Prince R, Allen FN, Farrar JT (1970) Inhibitory beta-adrenergic receptors in the human distal esophagus. Am J Dig Dis 15:303-310

27. Di Marino AJ Jr, Cohen S (1982) Effect of an oral beta-2-adrenergic agonist on lower esophageal sphincter pressure in normals and in patients with achalasis. Dig Dis Sci 27:1063-1066

28. Boyle JT, Tuchman DN, Altschuler SM, et al (1985) Mechanisms for the association of gastroesophageal reflux and bronchospasm. Am Rev Respir Dis 131(Suppl):S16-S20

29. Moote DW, Lloyd DA, McCourtie DR, Wells GA (1986) Increase in gastroesophageal reflux during methacholine-induced bronchospasm. J Allergy Clin Immunol 78:619-623

30. Michoud MC, Leduc T, Proulx F, et al (1991) Effect of salbutamol on gastroesophageal reflux in healthy volunteers and patients with asthma. J Allergy Clin Immunol 87:762-767

31. Schindlbeck NE, Hinrich C, Huber RM, Muller-Lissner SA (1988) Effects of albuterol (salbutamol) on esophageal motility and gastroesophageal reflux in healthy volunteers. JAMA 260:3156-3158

32. Eastwood GL, Castell DD, Higgs RH (1975) Experimental esophagitis in cats impairs lower esophageal sphincter pressure. Gastroenterology 69:146-153

33. Andrew BL (1956) The nervous control of the cervical esophagus of the rat during swallowing. J Physiol (Lond) 134:729-740

34. Mansfield LE, Hameister HH, Spaulding HS, Smith NJ, Glab N (1981) The role of the vagus nerve in airway narrowing caused by intraesophageal hydrochloric acid provocation and esophageal distention. Ann Allergy 47:431-434

35. Abraham WM, Baugh LE (1995) Animal models of asthma. In: Busse WW, Holgate ST (eds) Asthma and rhinitis. Blackwell Scientific, Boston, pp 961-977

36. Soler M, Sielczak MW, Abraham WM (1989) A PAF-antagonist blocks antigen-induced airway hyperresponsiveness and inflammation in sheep. J Appl Physiol 67:406-413

Clinical Signs of Gastroesophageal Reflux

C. MICHELETTO[1], G. MIGLIARA[2], and S. TOGNELLA[1]

Introduction

Gastroesophageal reflux (GER) is a term used to refer to symptoms and events that result from abnormal regurgitation of gastric contents into the esophagus. GER can episodically occur in normal persons without provoking any complaint, thus representing a disorder that can commonly affect large segments of the general population. Untreated pathological GER impairs quality of life and can frequently lead to esophagitis or occasionally to Barrett's esophagus (with its tendency to become malignant). However, the spectrum of problems associated with GER has expanded to extra-esophageal sites [1, 2].

GER has long been regarded as a factor favoring the onset of respiratory disorders such as cough, hypersecretion, and wheezing (particularly nocturnal wheezing) [3-6]. Moreover, several investigators have emphasized the role of GER in increasing the risk for chronic respiratory diseases (e.g. bronchial asthma, chronic bronchitis, recurrent pneumonia, pulmonary fibrosis) [4, 7, 8].

The dominant complaints of GER patients are usually related to the upper gastrointestinal tract, but patients with reflux are also susceptible to the so-called atypical or extra-esophageal manifestations [9, 10], such as unexplained chest pain, hoarseness, chronic cough, and bronchoconstriction. Extra-esophageal manifestations can also occur when typical GER symptoms are minimal or absent. Two retrospective studies published in the 1960s introduced the concept of "silent GER" to describe patients with respiratory complications due to GER, without any typical gastroenterological symptom of GER [3, 11].

Typical Signs of GER

Common clinical symptoms of GER are heartburn, acid regurgitation, and dysphagia. Heartburn (or pyrosis) is experienced as a retrosternal sensation of

[1]Lung Department, Bussolengo General Hospital, Bussolengo (Verona), Italy; [2]Division of Bronchopneumology, IRCCS Ospedale Maggiore, Milan, Italy

burning and discomfort. Heartburn is a commonly used, but frequently misunderstood, term as it is sometimes used by patients to indicate indigestion, acid regurgitation, sour stomach, or "bitter belching". The terms burning, hot, or acid are typically used by patients unless the discomfort of heartburn becomes so intense that pain is experienced. Heartburn, the classic manifestation of GER, is probably the most common gastrointestinal complaint in the Western population: some surveys on American populations revealed that 33%-44% of subjects refer the occurence of heartburn at least monthly, and 7%-13% may have daily GER symptoms [12, 13].

Heartburn is predictably aggravated by multiple factors, particularly food (Table 1). Thus, it is frequently noted within one hour after eating, particularly following the largest meal of the day. Foods high in fat, sugars, chocolate, onion or carminatives may aggravate heartburn by decreasing the lower esophageal sphincter pressure [14]. Other foods, such as citrus products, are direct irritants to the inflamed esophageal mucosa: this mechanism is independent of pH and probably related to high osmolarity [15, 16].

Table 1. Food and drugs triggering digestive symptoms of GER

	Decrease of LES pressure	**Direct mucosal irritation**
Foods	Fat	Citrus products
	Sugar	Tomato-based products
	Chocolate	Spicy foods
	Onions	Apples
	Carminatives	Coffee
	Coffee	
	Tea	
	Licorice	
	Alcohol	
Medications	Progesterone	Aspirin
	Theophylline	NSAIDs
	Anticholinergic agents	Tetracycline
	α-Adrenergic antagonists	Quinidine
	Diazepam	Potassium chloride tablets
	Meperidine	Iron salts
	Nitrates	
	Calcium channel blockers	

LES, lower esophageal spincter; *NSAIDs*, nonsteroid anti-inflammatory drugs

Maneuvers that increase intra-abdominal pressure, including bending over, straining at defecation, lifting heavy objects, and performing isometric exercises may also aggravate heartburn. Emotions such as anxiety, fear, and worry may exacerbate heartburn probably by the amplification of symptoms rather than by a true increase in the amount of acid reflux [12, 17]. Heartburn may be accompanied by the appearance of fluid together with bitter acidic material, or salty fluid in the mouth.

Regurgitation describes the complaint of a bitter acid fluid in the mouth that commonly occurs at night or when bending over. It is important to distinguish regurgitation from vomiting: the absence of nausea, retching, and abdominal contractions should better suggest the occurence of regurgitation rather than vomiting. The coexistence of heartburn and acid regurgitation as dominant complaints corresponds to active GER, as defined by prolonged esophageal pH monitoring, a technique which is 78% sensitive and 60% specific [18].

Dysphagia, from the Greek *phagia* (to eat) and *dys* (difficulty, disordered), refers to the sensation of food being hindered in its normal passage from the mouth to the stomach. Most patients say that food "sticks", "hangs up", or "stops", or that they feel "the food just won't go down right". Dysphagia is experienced immediately after swallowing: when this sensation is unrelated to swallowing it should suggest the presence of a foreign body or globus, and should not be confused with dysphagia.

Atypical Signs of GER

Other symptoms of reflux disease include water brush, globus sensation, and, rarely, odynophagia. Water brush, or hypersalivation, is a relatively unusual symptom of GER in which patients can literally foam at the mounth, secreting as much as 10 ml saliva per minute. Water brush is induced by acid reflux, wherein esophageal acidification triggers an esophagosalivary reflex [19]. Although increased salivation accompanies acid reflux in most patients, it can be sometimes markedly exaggerated.

Globus sensation is the almost constant perception of a lump in the throat, irrespective of swallowing. Up to 46% of the general population has experienced the globus sensation at one time or another [20]: this particular sensation accounts for 3% of consultations to throat specialists [21], predominantly by middle-aged women. Despite the tendency to attribute globus to increased upper esophageal sphincter pressure as a result of esophageal acidification, this hypothesis is not yet confirmed experimentally [22, 23].

Odynophagia (pain with swallowing) is an extremely unusual symptom of GER, being far more typical of infectious esophagitis or pill ulceration. The cases of GER in which odynophagia is prominent are usually associated with an esophageal ulcer or deep erosions.

Angina-like retrosternal chest pain is not always caused by cardiac disease, as reported by several studies of esophageal monitoring in patients with noncardiac chest pain [24-27]. The proportion of patients in whom there was a significant correlation between esophageal abnormalities and pain varied from 12% to 90%; these figures depend on the differences, sometimes substantial, in the criteria used for both patient selection and instrumental diagnostic indicators.

Respiratory Signs of GER

Up to 10% of patients with GER refer pulmonary symptoms due to gastric regurgitation [28]. It is generally recognized that GER may be an important cause of respiratory disorders, particularly intrinsic asthma, both in children and adults (Table 2).

Over the past 30 years, several papers (mainly based on clinical observations) drove the attention to the relationship between GER and asthma [1, 2, 12, 29-31], as analytically reported in the chapter by Dal Negro and Turco in the present volume. The reasons for these concurrent pathological events are not yet fully understood: whether reflux by itself initiates or exacerbates asthma, or whether asthma by itself (or its treatment) may primarily cause GER is still debated [3, 32-35]. However, several clinical studies estimated that GER occurs three-times more frequently in asthma patients than in the general population, and has a prevalence of 30%-89% in asthma patients [3-5, 28, 33, 36]. More recently, about three-fourths of asthmatics have been described as having acid GER, increased frequency of reflux episodes, or heartburn independently of the use of bronchodilators, and reflux esophagitis was proved in about 40% [37].

Patients with GER-associated asthma (or possibly asthma due to GER) may manifest classic or atypical symptoms of GER, but approximately 25%-30% have clinically silent GER [38]. Additional symptoms suggestive of GER include dysphagia, odynophagia, atypical chest pain, and symptoms referred to the upper respiratory tract, or oropharynx. Nocturnal asthma, or the development of nocturnal coughing, choking, wheezing, or hoarseness on awakening should

Table 2. Respiratory signs and potential pulmonary manifestations of GER

Respiratory signs of GER

Hoarseness, especially in the morning
Repeated need to clear the throat
Sensation of pressure deep in the throat
Chronic persistent cough
Nocturnal or early morning wheezing
Hyperventilation
Laryngeal spasm

Potential pulmonary manifestations

Chronic asthma
Bronchitis
Bronchiectasis
Aspiration pneumonia
Atelectasis
Pulmonary fibrosis
Laryngitis

suggest GER during sleep [39]. Moreover, asthma symptoms may worsen following events known to aggravate GER, including meals, alcohol ingestion, and reclining. A recent study in which patients were asked if their asthma worsened following alcohol ingestion, large meals and recumbency confirmed that these situations caused asthma impairment in 4%, 39% and 21% of cases, respectively, while only 7.6% experienced a worsening of asthma following coffee assumption.

At present, ambulatory intraesophageal pH monitoring represents the gold standard for the diagnosis of pathologic GER [40], also because it facilitates investigating the possible relationship between GER episodes and wheezing, or other symptoms which are suggestive of bronchospasm. Pulmonary symptoms developing either during or immediately after (within 10 min) an episode of acid GER (i.e. esophageal pH < 4) are considered strictly related and suggestive for GER involvement in triggering respiratory symptoms [41, 42]. Prolonged pH monitoring performed by Sontag and coworkers in 48 consecutive adult asthmatics demonstrated that out of 142 episodes of wheezing, 15.5% and 9.9% occurred during or after GER, respectively, while 20.4% preceded GER [42].

GER patients who subsequently also prove to have asthma may present cough rather than symptoms of wheezing and breathlessness: Irwin et al. reported that chronic persistent cough (CPC), lasting from several months to years, can be the sole presenting manifestation of GER, so confirming that GER is clinically "silent" in 75% of patients studied [43]. Furthermore, they found that cough most commonly was due to one of four disorders (post-nasal drip syndrome, asthma, chronic bronchitis and gastroesophageal reflux) (Table 3), and that cough was primarily due to a single cause (82%), even though it can sometimes be the response to dual causes (18%) [44].

Table 3. Causes of chronic persistent cough. (Modified from [44])

Cause	Frequency (%)
Post-nasal drip syndrome	41
Asthma	24
Gastroesophageal reflux disease	21
Chronic bronchitis	5
Miscellaneous[a]	9

[a]Includes: bronchiectasis, bronchogenic carcinoma, left ventricular failure, sarcoidosis, and drug-induced cough

GER patients may also complain of a distinct set of clinical manifestations, which include persistent, nonproductive cough, accompanied by hoarseness, sensation of pressure deep in the throat, and continual need to clear the throat [45, 46]: also in this case the classic digestive symptoms of GER can often be minimal or absent. As discussed in this volume by Filiaci et al., the larynx is reported to be one possible target for reflux and it may produce symptoms when irritated by contact with gastric contents. Acid laryngitis has been recognized as a primary disorder and often presents with symptoms related to the throat [47]. In some patients with this constellation of symptoms, endoscopy shows a posterior laryngitis, even though some patients show a normal-appearing larynx, just as some patients with serious symptoms of reflux have a normal-appearing esophageal mucosa [45]. Furthermore, laryngeal sensitivity to refluxed gastric acid resulting in apnea, laryngospasm and respiratory arrest might be responsible for sudden infant death syndrome [48]. Another study suggested that chemoreceptors in the esophagus and pharynx, which are sensitized by acid gastric reflux, might respond to stimulation by causing apnea [49]. In this report, no less than 57% of infants studied had apnea after adequate medical antireflux therapy; the 43% who did not respond adequately to medical management had good results with antireflux surgery. Awake apnea in infants has also been attributed to GER, as described by Spitzer et al. [50]. Awake apnea, which generally occurs within one hour of feeding, is described as a sudden startled, or staring, expression and rigid posturing with subsequent hypotonia. Movements that predispose to GER, such as sudden flexing of the legs on the changing table or movement from a lying to sitting position, often precipitate symptoms of awake apnea [50].

More recently, Smyrnios and coworkers reported that post-nasal drip syndrome together with gastroesophageal reflux disease and asthma were the most common causes of CPC, accounting for 85% of all causes found [51]. Furthermore, they described the clinical picture of patients with cough attributable to GER disease: this kind of patient has disturbing cough lasting at least 3 weeks, does not smoke, does not take angiotensin-converting enzyme inhibitors, does not respond to therapy for post-nasal drip syndrome or asthma, and has normal or nearly normal chest radiograph findings [51]. Moreover, evaluation of the atopic condition can be a helpful discriminating indicator in building up the "identikit" of the asthmatic patient with GER.

Recently, our group carried out a study to investigate the primitive pathogenetic role of GER in asthma, and to assess specificity and sensitivity for both clinical signs and instrumental parameters currently used for checking GER. Even though the effect of atopy was negligible per se, intrinsic asthmatics were systematically older and characterized by a much later onset of their asthma (i.e. in their fifth decade of life), while atopic asthmatics were always younger (by about 15 years) with a much longer history of asthma (i.e. since their youth). Furthermore, while in atopic asthma the onset of respiratory symptoms always preceded the occurrence of specific digestive signs by several years, digestive symptoms occurred much earlier (more than 6 years) in a large proportion of nonatopic asthmatics. The pharmacological history of asthma patients with GER can also provide some interesting suggestions. In our study, from the pharmacological point of view, intrinsic asthmatics were the "more treated", probably because the conventional anti-asthma therapy (which is usually effective in atopic asthmatics) is less effective in these patients or, at least, because the control of their asthma is much more difficult. Moreover, long-term oral theophylline, which should be avoided in such cases because of its GER-inducing activity [52], is instead used twice daily in atopic asthmatics, emphasizing the iatrogenic potentialities of this respiratory drug in inducing GER [4, 8].

Many studies have emphasized that both kind and duration of digestive GER signs are not strictly related to the severity of structural esophageal lesions due to GER. In fact, the mechanisms involved in the development of all symptoms due to reflux are poorly understood. Several questions concerning the symptom perception in GER remain unanswered: it is not known, for instance, why some patients have heartburn whereas others, with apparently similar reflux patterns, do not. It was suggested that in patients with classic digestive GER, symptoms perception depends on the duration of acid exposure and on the upstream extension of acid refluxate [53].

Furthermore, it is also difficult to establish the relationship between extra-esophageal manifestations and digestive signs of GER, because these symptoms are often present in patients with normal biopsies from esophageal mucosa. The pathogenesis and pathophysiology of GER, such as the mechanisms by which intra-esophageal acid regurgitation from the stomach produces respiratory symptoms (particularly cough and bronchoconstriction) and the occurrence of esophagobronchial vagal reflexes, are still subjects of much debate. Acid reflux can also lead to heightened bronchial reactivity, as well as to microaspiration into both the larynx and upper airway [54].

Conclusions

Respiratory manifestations of GER are always challenging and sometimes represent the only presenting syndrome of GER disease. A vagally mediated reflex has been described in GER-associated cough, while acid-related asthma is still a complex puzzle among vagally mediated reflexes, airway hypersensitivity, and microaspiration into airways.

When GER is not suspected as a cause or as a trigger of the pulmonary signs of asthma, the medical management can sometimes result unsatisfactory and the patient's respiratory disease can frequently be considered refractory to any conventional respiratory treatment.

Further work is needed to evaluate the cost-effectiveness of diagnosing and treating these patients. Nevertheless, all patients with persistent or difficult-to-treat asthma (particularly intrinsic asthma) should also be extensively investigated for the underlying GER-related pathogenesis of their asthma.

References

1. Richter JE, Castell DO (1982) Gastroesophageal reflux pathogenesis, diagnosis and therapy. Ann Intern Med 97:93-103
2. Deschner WK, Benjamin SB (1989) Extraesophageal manifestations of gastro-esophageal reflux disease. Am J Gastroenterol 84:1-5
3. Kennedy JH (1962) "Silent" gastro-esophageal reflux: an important but little known cause of pulmonary complications. Dis Chest 42:42-45
4. Mays EE (1976) Intrinsic asthma in adults associated with gastroesophageal reflux. JAMA 236:2626-2628
5. Sontag SJ, O'Connel S, Khandelwal S, et al (1990) Most asthmatics have gastro-esophageal reflux with or without bronchodilator therapy. Gastroenterology 99:613-620
6. Ekstrom T, Tibbling L (1988) Gastroesophageal reflux and nocturnal asthma. Eur Respir J 1:636-638
7. Belsey R (1960) The pulmonary complications of esophageal disease. Br J Dis Chest 54:342-345
8. Clemencon GH, Osterman PO (1961) Hiatal hernia in bronchial asthma: the impor-tance of concomitant pulmonary emphysema. Gastroenterolgy 95:110-120
9. Gastal OL, Castell JA, Castell DO (1994) Frequency and site of gastroesophageal reflux in patients with chest symptoms. Chest 106:1793-1796
10. Barish CF, Wu WC, Castell DO (1985) Respiratory complication of gastroesophageal reflux. Arch Intern Med 145:1882-1888
11. Urschel HR, Paulson DL (1967) Gastroesophageal reflux and hiatal hernia: compli-cations of therapy. J Thorac Cardiovasc Surg 53:21-25
12. A Gallup survey on heartburn across America (1988) The Gallup Organization, Princeton NJ, p 28
13. Nebel OT, Fornes MF, Castell DO (1976) Symptomatic gastroesophageal reflux: inci-dence and precipitating factors Dig Dis Sci 21:953-956
14. Richter JE, Castell DO (1981) Drugs, food and other substances in the cause and treatment of reflux esophagitis. Med Clin North Am 65:1223-1234
15. Price SF, Smithson KW, Castell DO (1988) Food sensitivity in reflux esophagitis. Gastroenterology 75:240-245
16. Lloyd DA, Borda IT (1988) Food-induced heartburn: effect of osmolarity. Gastroenterology 80:740-746
17. Pulliam TJ, Bradley LA, Dalton CB, et al (1989) The role of psychological stress in gastroesophageal reflux disease. Gastroenterology 96:A208
18. Klauser AG, Schindlebeck NE, Muller-Lissner SA (1990) Symptoms in gastro-oesophageal reflux disease. Lancet 335:205-208
19. Helm JF, Dodds WJ, Hogan WJ (1987) Salivary response to esophageal acid in nor-mal subjects and patients with reflux esophagitis. Gastroenterology 92:1393-1397
20. Thompson WA, Heaton KW (1982) Heartburn and globus in apparently healthy people. Can Med Assoc J 126:46-48
21. Thompson WG (1989) Gut reactions. Plenum, New York, p 93
22. Kahrilas PJ, Dodds WJ, Dent J, et al (1987) The effect of sleep, spontaneous gastro-esophageal reflux and a meal on UES pressure in humans. Gastroenterology 92:466-471
23. Vakil NB, Kahrilas PJ, Dodds WJ, et al (1989) Absence of an upper esophageal sphincter response to acid reflux. Am J Gastroenterol 84:606-610
24. Voskuil JH, Cramer MJ, Breumelhof R, et al (1996) Prevalence of esophageal disorders in patients with chest pain newly referred to the cardiologist. Chest 109:1210-1214

25. Soffer EE, Scalabrini P, Wingate DC (1989) Spontaneous noncardiac chest pain: value of ambulatory esophageal pH monitoring. Dig Dis Sci 34:1651-1655

26. Wu WC, Castell DO, Richter JE (1988) Spontaneous noncardiac chest pain: evaluation by 24-h ambulatory esophageal motility and pH monitoring. Gastroenterology 94:878-886

27. Lam HG, Dekker W, Kan G, et al (1992) Acute noncardiac chest pain in a coronary unit. Evaluation by 24-h pressure and pH recording of the esophagus. Gastroenterology 102:453-460

28. Davis MV (1972) Relationship between pulmonary disease, hiatal hernia, and gastroesophageal reflux. N Y State J Med 72:935-938

29. Nebel OT, Fornes MF, Castell DO (1976) Symptomatic gastroesophageal reflux: incidence and precipitating factors. Dig Dis Sci 21:953-956

30. Irwin RS, French CL, Curley FJ, et al (1993) Chronic cough due to gastroesophageal reflux: clinical, diagnostic and pathogenic aspects. Chest 104:1511-1517

31. Harding SM, Richter JE (1992) Gastroesophageal reflux disease and asthma. Semin Gastrointest Dis 3:139-150

32. Allen CJ, Newhouse MT (1984) Gastroesophageal reflux and chronic respiratory disease. Am Rev Respir Dis 129:645-647

33. Overholt RH, Ashraf MM (1966) Esophageal reflux as a trigger in asthma. N Y State J Med 66:3030-3032

34. Larrain A, Carrasco J, Galleguillos J, Pope CE II (1981) Reflux treatment improves lung function in patients with intrinsic asthma. Gastroenterology 80:1204 (abstract)

35. Ayres JG, Miles JF (1996) Oesophageal reflux and asthma. Eur Respir J 9:1073-1078

36. Mansfield LE (1989) Gastroesophageal reflux and asthma. Postgrad Med 86:265-269

37. Sontag SJ (1997) Gastroesophageal reflux and asthma. Am J Med 103:84S-90S

38. Simpson WG (1995) Gastroesophageal reflux disease and asthma. Arch Intern Med 155:798-803

39. Martin RT (1992) Nocturnal asthma. Clin Chest Med 13:533-550

40. Castell DO (1991) pH monitoring versus other tests for gastroesophageal reflux disease: is this the gold standard? In: Richter JE (ed) Ambulatory esophageal pH monitoring: practical approach and clinical applications. Igaku-Shoin Medical, New York, pp 101-113

41. Sontag SJ (1991) Pulmonary abnormalities and gastroesophageal reflux disease. In: Richter JE (ed) Ambulatory esophageal pH monitoring: practical approach and clinical applications. Igaku-Shoin Medical, New York, pp 151-166

42. Sontag S, O'Connel S, Klandelwal S, et al (1989) Does wheezing occur in association with an episode of gastroesophageal reflux? Gastroenterology 96:482

43. Irwin RS, French CL, Curley FJ, et al (1993) Chronic cough due to gastroesophageal reflux: clinical, diagnostic and pathogenetic aspects. Chest 104:1511-1517

44. Irwin RS, Curley FJ, French CL (1990) Chronic cough. Am Rev Respir Dis 141:640-647

45. Pope II CE (1994) Acid reflux disorders. New Engl J Med 331:656-660

46. Gaynor EB (1991) Otolaryngologic manifestations of gastroesophageal reflux. Am J Gastroenterol 86:801-808

47. Kambic V, Radsel Z (1984) Acid posterior laryngitis. J Laryngol Otol 98:1237-1240

48. Foglia RP, Fonkalsrud EW, Ament E, et al (1980) Gastroesophageal fundoplication for the management of chronic pulmonary disease in children. Am J Surg 140:72-79

49. Herbst JJ, Minton SD, Books LS (1979) Gastroesophageal reflux causing respiratory distress and apnea in newborn infants. J Pediatr 95:763-768

50. Spitzer AR, Boyle JT, Tuchmann DN, et al (1984) Awake apnea associated with gastroesophageal reflux: a specific clinical syndrome. J Pediatr 104:200-205

51. Smyrnios NA, Irwin RS, Curley FJ, French CL (1998) From a prospective study of chronic cough: diagnostic and therapeutic aspects in older adults. Arch Intern Med 158:1222-1228
52. Hubert D, Gaudric M, Guerre J, et al (1988) Effect of theophylline on gastroesophageal reflux patients with asthma. J Allergy Clin Immunol 81:1168-1174
53. Weusten BLAM, Akkermans LMA, Gerard P, et al (1995) Symptoms perception in gastroesophageal reflux disease is dependent on spatiotemporal reflux characteristics. Gastroenterology 108:1739-1744
54. Harding SM, Richter JE (1997) The role of gastroesophageal reflux in chronic cough and asthma. Chest 111:1389-1402

Epidemiology of Gastroesophageal Reflux in Asthma

R.W. Dal Negro and P. Turco

Introduction

Gastroesophageal reflux (GER) represents a well-established digestive disorder which was identified by gastroenterologists long ago. Hypothesis of the occurrence of GER-related respiratory complications, particularly asthma symptoms, was frequently regarded with scepticism in the past. Similarly, respiratory complications of GER were only seen as negligible clinical suggestions.

More recently, even though the coexistence of GER and bronchial asthma has been progressively accepted in general terms, the critical point still impending is to assess whether GER per se can lead to bronchial asthma or conversely, whether bronchial asthma can induce GER. In other words, despite the occasional combination of GER and respiratory signs (such as recurrent cough, wheezing, shortness of breath, nocturnal dyspnea, hyperventilation or apnea episodes) a possible causative role of GER in the genesis or aggravation of asthma still represents the most relevant and difficult subject to clarify.

This particular topic represents a very complex puzzle indeed, which was approached individually by several medical disciplines (such as surgery, pediatrics, gastroenterology, pneumology) in the past decades in order to assess the relative role of all different pathogenetic factors involved. Many studies have been conducted, but merging the different backgrounds with the aim to build-up and share common knowledge was attempted only in recent years: the cultural basis of this neglected, but still challanging, matter of research has then been enriched substantially in a short time.

Clinical contributions on the occurrence of bronchial asthma in GER patients have become more frequent, and even more frequent are the attempts to correlate the pathophysiological situation of these subjects from both the gastroenterological and pneumological points of view. Furthermore, biologists and neurophysiologists are contributing greatly to a more precise definition of the events which characterize bronchial asthma and GER when combined. The new pathophysiological evidence has led to the present pathogenetic theories.

Lung Department, Bussolengo General Hospital, Bussolengo (Verona), Italy

Also, the development of specific technologies greatly facilitates the characterization of these patients, so that epidemiological investigations focusing on the prevalence of GER-induced respiratory disorders are now possible.

Old Clinical Studies

In 1892, Sir W. Osler observed that asthma patients do not usually have dinner to avoid the occurrence of nocturnal wheezing and awakenings [1]. At that time, the frequent concomitance of respiratory and digestive problems had been known for a few years following a case report concerning a subject with a dilated esophagus [2].

During the first decades of the present century, the occurrence of respiratory signs was clinically described in more than 10% of subjects presenting esophageal dysfunction such as achalasia [3]. The occurrence of asthma-like syndromes was also documented during intraoperative anesthesia for obstetric surgery, because pulmonary aspiration of gastric contents was the only mechanism suggested to explain the onset of the pulmonary events [4].

More than 10 years later, further important observations were made concerning the incidence of hiatal hernia in asthma patients when presenting GER. In these circumstances, the critical role of asthma in determining or promoting GER was underlined: it was mainly related to the asthma-induced lung hyperinflation and to the subsequent development of increased intrathoracic pressure [5]. This contribution still represents the first important attempt to link some clinical observations to the underlying pathophysiology. In other words, a few simple clinical signs were transformed into an organized and logical pathogenetic theory, which could easily explain the coexistence of bronchial asthma and GER.

After a decade, this hypothesis was confirmed by a paper which reported that hiatal hernia was also more frequent in asthmatic children with GER than in nonasthmatic children [6]. Moreover, it was also found that the radiological severity of GER was related to the clinical severity of respiratory disorders observed in these children. This peculiar aspect had been previously studied in adults. The incidence of hiatal hernia was in fact increased during long-lasting intrinsic asthma, and respiratory symptoms of these subjects were significantly reduced by non-specific antireflux therapy [7]. In this study the possible link between intrinsic asthma and GER was clearly mentioned and suggested for the first time.

All this clinical evidence on the association between bronchial asthma and GER greatly contributed to augment the interest in this peculiar nosological entity, but the real dimension of the problem still remained to be defined in epidemiological terms. The poor epidemiological approach gave a true bias to the majority of clinical studies. Usually, clinical and parametrical criteria for measuring and defining bronchial asthma (such as etiology, severity, duration, and therapy) and GER (such as extent, rhythm and frequency of episodes, duration, body position for its occurrence, dependency on meals and degree of acidity) were not declared previously and precisely in these investigational protocols, and the unique indicators used were only conventional clinical signs and/or radiological findings. Nevertheless, the first pathophysiological suggestions were based on these pivotal studies of bronchial asthma and GER, which more or less supported the rationale for the future specific experimentation.

Other more complex investigations a few years later led to further substantial increases in the specific knowledge. New technologies and diagnostic equipment consented the measurement of new functional parameters which proved important in assessing pulmonary and digestive pathological events in these circumstances, with high degree of sensitivity and specificity.

At the end of the 1960s, further studies drew attention to the frequent occurrence of asthmatic respiratory signs (i.e. wheezing) in GER patients. Most of these contributions reported some outcome which mainly derived from surgical experiences. In fact, the beneficial effects of the antireflux surgical approach were particularly underlined in these studies [8-10]. Most of these clinical investigations proved limited and failed in assessing the effective prevalence of asthma in GER subjects. In particular, the cause-effect relationship between the events was not sufficiently focused, because once again the epidemiological approach to the problem was poor, namely in terms of insufficient definition of both asthma and GER severity, unclear preliminary identification of confounding factors such as smoking and atopy, and insuffecent precision in patient inclusion and exclusion criteria.

In 1976, a true increased prevalence of GER in adult asthma patients (smokers and nonsmokers) was assessed, and the higher frequency of GER in intrinsic asthma was particularly emphasized [7]. These results were confirmed in pediatric patients by a controlled study designed to investigate the prevalence and causative role of GER in children (such as in absence of active cigarette smoking, a likely confounding factor) with obstructive bronchitis [11].

In the 1980s, other studies reinforced these previous suggestions: the high frequency of GER in asthma patients received further confirmation, and a prevalence of 30%-65% was reported in different studies [12-15]. Unfortunately, most of these studies were poorly controlled and the evaluation of respiratory function was frequently inadequate. However, the cultural interest was greatly emphasized on this topic, and several, more controlled investigations were subsequently initiated.

Recent Controlled Studies

At the end of the last decade, the frequency of GER was investigated for the first time in a sample of consecutive asthma patients according to a random design, and both spirometrical and esophageal pH measurements were carried out for 4 hours in all subjects [16]. The prevalence of GER was 32% in this study, but no correlation at all was proved between forced expiratory volume in 1 s (FEV_1)

changes and variations of different parameters deriving from the esophageal pH monitoring, particularly in severe asthma.

Other studies compared the incidence of GER in asthmatics and in the normal population: figures varied between 30%-89%, and a consensus was reached around 50%. All age groups were affected equally, and the combination with bronchial asthma proved particularly evident in children who have GER more frequently. Thus, the pathogenetic role of the long-term contact of acidic gastric content with esophageal structures was underlined [17].

The clinical relevance of GER on the natural history of asthma was questioned by Ekstrom and Tibbling [18] who did not show any causal relationship between the documented GER episodes and the onset of asthma symptoms, peak expiratory flow rate (PEFR) changes, or daily use of bronchodilators in a sample of subjects affected by GER and moderate to severe asthma. However, a statistically significant, even though small, drop in FEV_1 values during acid perfusion of the esophagus was measured in these subjects [18].

When, further to the simplistic description of clinical signs, some reproducible indicators of gastroenterological function were introduced to assess the limits of GER abnormality (such as the parameters used in 24-hour gastro-esophageal pH monitoring), 81.8% of asthmatics showed pathological episodes of GER. Of these, 25% had only upright acid reflux, 10.6% had only supine acid reflux, and 46.2% had combined upright and supine reflux episodes, without any difference in age, cigarette smoking habit, and alcohol or bronchodilators consumption [19]. The high prevalence of GER indicated by this study could lead to some incorrect assumptions, because all recruited patients had been previously selected on basis of their consolidated history of digestive signs (i.e. of GER). In other words, the population investigated in this study did not reflect the true condition of all asthmatics at all, but only of those subjects already experiencing some of the most specific signs of GER for a long time. The true epidemiology of this peculiar pathological condition still remained a field open for investigation because data proved once again difficult to obtain and interpret.

Esophageal pH monitoring has been employed in several studies which contributed to support [20-22] or refute [18, 23, 24] the hypothesis of GER-related asthma.

In 1994, our group investigated the prevalence of GER in a sample of consecutive, well matched, adult mild asthmatics who were recruited over a 6-month period according to a random model which eliminated the most relevant confounding factors (e.g. regular hormonal treatment in women, occupational risks, and cigarette smoking). In this study, the prevalence of GER was for the first time assessed separately in atopic (elevated total IgE, positive prick test and radioallergosorbent test, RAST) and nonatopic (low total IgE, negative prick test and RAST) subjects, in order to evaluate the potential role of atopy in the combination of asthma and GER [25].

In all subjects, asthma severity was assessed according to clinical and spirometrical criteria, previously standardized. Criteria for the definition of pathological GER were barium contrast radiology, digestive endoscopy, and gastroesophageal 24-hour pH monitoring, and the functional indices of DeMeester et al. were assumed [26]. Sensitivity and specificity of these indicators, and of the most common clinical signs of GER (e.g. acid regurgitation, heartburn, and chest pain) were also calculated together with the prevalence of hiatal hernia in the two subsets of subjects.

Atopic asthmatics were significantly younger (mean age 38.0 vs. 53.2 years, $p < 0.007$), and had a longer history of asthma than nonatopic subjects in whom asthma systematically starts at a later age. Moreover, in atopic subjects asthma onset always preceded the onset of digestive signs of GER by an average of 6 years, while in 47% of intrinsic asthmatics the onset of GER symptoms preceded that of asthma by an average of 7 years: in these cases the primitive role of GER in the pathogenesis of asthma was greatly emphasized. A further substantial contribution to this suggestion can be obtained by considering that the prevalence of hiatal hernia was much higher in intrinsic than in atopic asthmatics (38.9% and 15.8%, respectively; ratio 2.5).

In our experience, the global prevalence of GER was confirmed to be high indeed (80%), ranging from 78.9% in atopic to 83.3% in nonatopic subjects. No significant correlation between duration of digestive symptoms and extent of bronchial obstruction was found in our study. From this point of view, the pulmonary dysfunction (equally mild) which was originally assessed in all subjects recruited for the study could be regarded as a potential bias.

Some of our results, particularly those concerning intrinsic asthmatics, tend to confirm an older investigation in which 46% of intrinsic adult asthmatics (but only 5% of normal controls) were found to have GER, as verified by means of barium contrast radiology only [7]. The lower percentage of subjects with pathological GER as reported in this previous study is likely due to the different, and much less sensitive, diagnostic method utilized more than two decades ago to assess GER in asthma patients. Also in our study, the 24-hour pH monitoring was confirmed to be the most sensitive method for GER investigation, much more than both gastroesophageal endoscopy and radiology. This is likely because acid regurgitation and heartburn are the most specific signs for the clinical identification of GER [25, 26].

A similarly high prevalence of GER in asthma was calculated in an endoscopic study of 182 consecutive adult asthmatics, in which 43% of patients had morphological evidence of esophagitis [27]. In particular, when the method for assessing abnormality of GER episodes was 24-hour esophageal pH monitoring, 82% of asthmatics showed abnormal amounts of acid reflux [19].Therefore, the crucial outcomes of our epidemiological investigation were confirmed and highlighted [25].

Quite recently, the prevalence of GER symptoms was also evaluated in asthmatics and in controls by means of a questionnaire: 77% of asthma patients experienced heartburn, 55% acid regurgitation, and 24% swallowing difficulties [28]. In the week prior to completing the questionnaire, 41% of asthmatics had GER-associated respiratory signs, and 28% used respiratory drugs to control asthma symptoms while experiencing GER [28, 29].

A further confirmation, indirect in this case, of the active role of GER in triggering or causing asthma derives from several studies, all proving that aggressive acid suppression may improve asthma symptoms significantly, or decrease the need for bronchodilators or steroids in 75% of patients [30, 31].

Finally in comparison to atopic asthma patients, intrinsic asthmatics included in our study showed a curious pharmaco-epidemiological outcome which has never been described previously: their therapeutic regimen was more complex indeed, and they were much more frequently (ratio 2:1) treated with oral theophylline, which is a well known GER-inducing substance [32-34].

Conclusions

Epidemiological studies, together with specific clinical and pharmacological trials carried out recently, showed that acid GER and asthma can coexist in a large proportion of asthmatics, particularly in intrinsic asthma patients. Distal esophagitis is present in 30%-40% of these cases.

Even though the causative role of GER in asthma has not yet been clarified exhaustively, the problem of GER and asthma combination can no longer be neglected, neither in clinical nor in pathophysiological terms, particularly in difficult-to-treat chronic asthma.

References

1. Osler WB (1892) The principles of medicine. Appleton, NewYork
2. Mermod E (1887) Dilatation diffuse de l'oesophage. Rev Med Suisse Rom, quoted in N Engl J Med 245:441
3. Vinson EP (1924) Diagnosis and treatment of cardiospasm. JAMA 82:859-863
4. Mendelson CL (1946) The aspiration of stomach contents into the lungs during obstetric anesthesia. Am J Obstet Gynecol 52:191-194
5. Clemecon GH, Sterman P (1961) Hiatal hernia in bronchial asthma: the importance of concomitant pulmonary emphysema. Gastroenterology 95:110-115
6. Darling DB, McCauley RGK, Leonidas JC, Schwartz AM (1978) Gastroesophageal reflux in infants and children: correlation of radiological severity and pulmonary pathology. Pediatr Radiol 127:735-740
7. Mays EE (1976) Intrinsic asthma in adults: association with gastroesophageal reflux. JAMA 236:2626-2628
8. Overholt RH, Ashraf MM (1966) Esophageal reflux as a trigger in asthma. N Y State J Med 66:3030-3032
9. Davis MV (1969) Evolving concepts regarding hiatal hernia and gastroenterological reflux. Ann Thorac Surg 1:120-123
10. Babb RR, Notarangelo J, Smith VM (1970) Wheezing: a clue to gastroenterological reflux. Am J Gastroenterol 53:230-233
11. Danus O, Cesar C, Larrain A, Pope II CE (1976) Esophageal reflux: an unrecognised cause of recurrent obstructive bronchitis in children. J Pediatr 89:220-224

12. Giudicelli R, Dupin B, Surpas P, et al (1990) Reflux gastro-esophagien et manifestations respiratoires: attitude diagnostique, indications thérapeutiques et résultats. Ann Chir 44:552-554

13. Pasquis P, Tardiff C, Nouvet G (1983) Reflux gastroesophagien et affections respiratoires. Bull Eur Physiopathol Resp 19:645-658

14. Perrin-Fayolle M, Bel A, Kofman J, et al (1980) Asthma et reflux gastro-esophagien: résultats d'une enquête portant sur 150 cas. Poumon Coeur 36:225-230

15. Ramon P, Mallart-Voisin A, Wallaert B, et al (1998) Association asthma et reflux gastroesophagien: stratégie des examens complémentaires. Rev Med Respir 2:289-294

16. Pin I, Cignoux C, Delmas-Vassort D, et al (1989) Relation chronologique entre reflux gastro-esophagien et asthma. Rev Mal Resp 6:255-260

17. Goldman JM, Bennet JR (1990) Gastro-esophageal reflux and asthma; a common association, but of what clinical importance? Gut 31:1-3

18. Ekstrom T, Tibbling L (1987) Gastroesophageal reflux and the triggering of bronchial asthma: negative report. Eur J Respir Dis 71:177-180

19. Sontag SJ, O'Connell S, Khandelwal S, et al (1990) Most asthmatics have gastroesophageal reflux with or without bronchodilator therapy. Gastroenterology 99:613-620

20. Mansfield LE, Stein MR (1978) Gastroesophageal reflux and asthma: a possible reflex mechanism. Ann Allergy 41:224-226

21. Pellegrini CA, DeMeester TR, Johnson LF, et al (1979) Gastroesophageal reflux and pulmonary aspiration: incidence, functional abnormality, and results of surgical therapy. Surgery 86:110-119

22. Hughes DM, Spier S, Rivlin J, Levison H (1983) Gastroesophageal reflux during sleep in asthmatic patients. J Pediatr 102:666-672

23. Donald IP, Ford GA, Wilkinson SP (1987) Is 24-hour ambulatory oesophageal pH monitoring useful in a district general hospital? Lancet 1:89-92

24. Jolley SG, Herbst JJ, Johnson DG, et al (1981) Esophageal pH monitoring during sleep identifies children with respiratory symptoms from gastroesophageal reflux. Gastroenterology 80:1501-1506

25. Pomari C, Micheletto C, Dal Negro R (1994) Bronchial asthma and gastroesophageal reflux: an epidemiological investigation. Preliminary results. Eur Respir J 7(Suppl 18):15

26. DeMeester TR, Wang C, Wesley JA, et al (1980) Technique, indications and clinical use of 24 hour esophageal monitoring. J Thorac Cardiovasc Surg 79:656-670

27. Sontag SJ, Underwood M, Brant R, et al (1992) Prevalence of esophagitis in asthmatics. Gut 33:872-876

28. Field SK, Underwood M, Brant R, et al (1996) Prevalence of gastroesophageal reflux symptoms in asthma. Chest 106:316-322

29. Irwin RS, Curley FJ, French CL (1993) Difficult-to-control asthma: contributing factors and outcome of a systematic management protocol. Chest 103:1662-1669

30. Harding SM, Richter JE (1997) The role of gastroesophageal reflux in chronic cough and asthma. Chest 111:1389-1402

31. Sontag SJ (1997) Gastroesophageal reflux and asthma. Am J Med 103:84s-90s

32. Goyal RK, Rattan S (1978) Neurohumoral, hormonal, and drug receptors for the lower esophageal sphincter. Gastroenterology 74:598-602

33. Stein MR, Towner TG, Weber RW, et al (1980) The effect of theophylline on the lower esophageal sphincter pressure. Ann Allergy 45:238-241

34. Berquist WE, Rachelefsky GS, Kadden M, et al (1981) Effect of theophylline on gastroesophageal reflux in normal adults. J Allergy Clin Immunol 67:407-411

Gastroesophageal Reflux and Nonspecific Hyperreactivity of Upper Aerodigestive Tract: Possible Correlations with Otorhinolaryngological Disorders

F. Filiaci, G. Zambetti, M. Luce, and R. Romeo

Introduction

Gastroesophageal reflux (GER), a common disorder of the upper digestive tract, is primarily caused by release of the lower esophageal sphincter associated with delayed gastric emptying, abnormal esophageal mucosal resistance, and increased irritative capacity of the refluxate [1]. A clinical classification divides GER into a typical form with the classic pyrosis and an atypical form [2]. Patients with respiratory symptoms fall into the latter atypical, or extraesophageal, form that characterizes the "silent" GER. [3]. In fact, the initial symptomatology is often characterized by a succession of symptoms (e.g. dysphagia, foreign body sensation, chronic throat clearing, hoarseness, cough, otalgia, obstructive apnea, and recurrent bronchitis and pneumonia) that suggest the direct involvement of the upper and lower airways.

The pathogenetic mechanisms in GER-associated respiratory symptoms may involve direct acid reflux, inducing mucosal damage to the upper airways and, possibly, organ injury. Alternatively, they may result from vagus nerve reflexes which lead to laryngospasm and bronchospasm without any direct involvement of acid in the upper airway mucosa [4-7]. In this regard, GER has recently been implicated in the pathophysiology of numerous otolaryngological conditions such as chronic pharyngitis and laryngitis, dysphagia, cough, hoarseness [8-11], carcinoma of the larynx [12], subglottic stenosis [13], and Reinke's edema [14]. Moreover, the association between asthma and GER is supported by many publications [15-17]. However, it remains to be determined whether asthma is a primary disorder or if it follows GER, and if reflux represents the initial problem or a secondary clinical picture due to other diseases.

Department of Otorhinolaryngology, University of Rome La Sapienza, Policlinico Umberto I, Rome, Italy

Considering the problem, we posed the following questions: "Why does esophageal acid reflux induce noxious injury in only the inferior one-third of the esophagus and on the larynx and pharynx?" For the association between upper and lower airways: "Can we hypothesize a common disorder that also involves the esophagus?" and "Why must we only consider the known pathologic succession of reflux (esophageal disorder, laryngeal/pharyngeal injury, tracheal-lower airways pathology) and not hypothesize hyperreactivity as the primary problem that with time could involve in succession the nose, pharynx, larynx, trachea, and inferior one-third of the esophagus?"

Physioanatomic Organization of the Upper Airways

The environmental air must be conditioned before it arrives in the lower airways, and this function is carried out by the nondeformable structures of the upper airways; these are, in order, the *nose, epipharynx, oropharynx* and *hypopharynx,* and *larynx,* or in complementary or vicarious breathing the *mouth, oropharynx, hypopharynx,* and *larynx.* Conditioning of air acts directly on temperature and humidity, and serves to prevent foreign particles or hydrosoluble gases from reaching delicate structures such as the alveoli. Air humidification occurs almost exclusively in the anterior portion of the nasal cavities (rich in serous glands) by the direct passage of water from the mucous to the air. Temperature conditioning is linked to the exchange of heat between arterial vessels (which in the nose are plentiful) and the air from the whirling movements and from the variations in volume of the turbinates (due to involvement of the cavernous bodies).

The filter function is carried out by structures (such as the turbinates) which form obstacles to the inspiratory air flow as they protrude into the respiratory space. These structures create vortices and currents increase the air contact with the mucosa, and thereby increase the possibility to stop foreign particles in the mucosal layer. Filtering occurs by (1) alternate anatomic contraction and dilatation which, using the variations in pressure and flux, trap the smaller particles in the narrowest sections; (2) a drop in pressure in the broader sections; and (3) sudden variations of direction in the pharyngeal and oropharyngeal cavities causing the air to meet the adenoid surface and leave corpuscular particles adhered to the mucous layer.

Most conditioning of the environmental air is done by the nasal-epipharynx. However, in oral breathing the larynx, representing the last barrier to particles, is obliged to replace the missing nasal functions.

Inflammation Induced by Hyperreactivity

The integrity of the mucous membrane as well as the rheologic properties of the mucous layer are considered to be of primary importance in the physiopathology of the nose, sinus, mouth, pharynx and larynx. Since the upper airways are priming territory in the organization of the nasal immunitary system (NALT), it is understandable that in normal conditions the local characteristics can vary according to the contingent needs (physiological reactivity). Problems arise if the local response is abnormal compared to the entity of the stimulus or, in contrast, if the response to a stronger than normal stimulus is insufficient; in this case hyperreactivity occurs. Such hyperreactivity is influenced by constitutional (besides the genetic predisposition) and environmental factors (e.g. pollution, additives, colorants, sulfur and nitrogen dioxides, ozone) through the following mechanisms:

1. Amplification of the activity of the connection system between exogenous normal stimuli and local responses by:
   (a) Diminishing tone of smooth perivasal and periglandular muscular fibroblasts;
   (b) Increase in the number of receptor sites (imbalance in favor of beta-2);
   (c) Variation in enzymatic inhibitors, leading to alteration in intracellular biochemical mechanisms.
2. Increase in the mechanisms which carry stimuli:
   (a) Increase in trigeminal and vagal efferent fibers;
   (b) Diminished stimulation threshold for mastocytes, eosinophils and neutrophils, leading to increased cell recruitment and increased production of mediators;
   (c) Increased nasal and pharyngeal epithelium permeability to irritants.
3. Modulation by the psychological status (e.g. frustration, sense of guilt, humiliation) leading to nasal hyperreactive symptomatology.

The possibility of an exchange of information between the immune and nervous systems is one of the most fascinating hypotheses relating to the mechanism of defense of the human body (including nasal reactivity). This is especially true considering that both the sensitive cortex and the subcortical structures, such as the reticular brain stem substances and the hypothalamus, have regulatory and modulatory roles on the different afferences and efferences which control vasomotricity and glandular secretion of the mucosa. Nasal-pharyngeal hyperreactivity is therefore able to cause local inflammation, with objective and subjective symptoms that may even be insignificant to the patient. The inflammation has an immunomediated component (dysregulation of cellular type) and a neurogenic component due to an imbalance between sympathetic and parasympathetic autonomic systems (with prevalence of the latter). Stimuli from cellular injury on congenitally hyperreactive fibers and on uncovered fibers result in a release of neuropeptides (for axon reflexes).

A physician who is called to cure the acute phase of a reaction must aim, above all, to avoid recurrence of inflammation. This is important because chronic and widespread inflammation leads to hypertrophy of the turbinates, nasal polyposis, irreversible hypertrophy of the adenoid tissue, chronic pharyngitis, Reinke's edema, asthma, and eventually noxious irreversible injury even if using surgical options. Amplification and self-maintenance of inflammation will arise from (1) recruiting and activation of eosinophil and neutrophil leukocytes followed by epithelial injury, (2) production of histamine-releasing factors from the basophil leukocytes, (3) release of leukotriene B4 (LTB4) and products of 15-lipo-oxygenase by eosinophils, and (4) activation of endothelial cells and fibroblasts.

Could the mechanism which induces inflammation after nasal hyperreactivity be extended to the upper digestive tract and to the esophagus? In our opinion the answer is affirmative, because in patients with only nasal disorders, oral breathing facilitates the contact of irritant substances with the uvulo-palatal-pharyngeal-laryngeal mucosa which is rich in vagal receptors.

Anatomy and Physiology of the Esophagus

The microscopic structure of the esophagus consists of: a pavement of stratified epithelium with its own lamina (with a lymphatic apparatus and serum-mucous glands); muscularis mucosae; submucosa which facilitates mucous flow and is rich in vessels; muscular layer (striatal fibers in the upper one-third and smooth fibers in the lower two-thirds); and peri-esophageal tissue in close contact (at the level of bronchial stricture) with the smooth musculature. This latter, in a longitudinal arrangement, completes the "C" of cartilaginous rings of the trachea. The macroscopic anatomy of the esophagus is characterized by cricoid (crico-pharyngeal muscle), bronchial and aortic strictures. These anatomical features are important because they show grounds for the onset and the maintenance of inflammation of neighboring organs due to direct contact with phlogistic mediators.

The progression of an alimentary bolus may be divided in three different but harmoniously integrated phases:
1. Oral phase (voluntary), characterized by chewing;
2. Pharyngeal phase (involuntary), stimulating the vagus nerve (from soft palate), the glosso-pharyngeal nerve (from posterior wall of the pharynx) and the superior laryngeal nerve (epiglottis). This results in raising of the soft palate, movement of the posterior pillars of the soft palate, closing of the laryngeal vestibule, and releasing of the superior and inferior sphincters.
3. Esophageal phase (involuntary):
   - Peristaltic wave for the progression of solid food;
   - Gravity strength for the progression of liquids.

At this point we can hypothesize that there may be more than one mechanism which determines the pathological reflux. Besides direct stimulation by hydrochloric acid, there may be a vagal reflex or, considering the anatomical lines between bronchi and esophagus, a direct release of phlogistic mediators to the esophagus. This condition worsenes and self-perpetuates the single pathologies (esophageal and bronchial) and results in non-specific inflammation due to the esophageal acid (second phase).

Considering that the nose, soft palate, trachea and esophagus all share vagal innervation (Table 1), and that the smooth musculature of the upper and lower airways as well as of the middle and lower esophagus are targets of the inflammation caused by non-specific hyperreactivity, we hypothesized that, in some "hyperreactive" subjects, irritating substances present in food could, during chewing or swallowing, stimulate a distal vagal reflex and, ultimately, the release of the lower esophageal sphincter. To our knowledge, this is the first report suggesting a role of upper airway hyperreactivity in the pathogenesis of GER disease that, in patients with congenital predisposition, could cause several clinical symptoms similar to allergies. On these grounds, we carried out a study of the possible relationship between GER and non-specific hyperreactivity of the upper airways.

Table 1. Vagus nerve innervation of upper and lower airways

Nerve fibers	Innervated organ or system
Motor	- Pharyngeal plexus - Muscles of velum palatinum and pharynx
Sensory	- External acoustic canal - Tympanic membrane - Maxillary sinus - Pharynx - Larynx - Cardiac plexus - Esophageal plexus - Bronchial plexus - Stomach - Liver - Solar plexus
Parasympathetic viscero-motor	- Ganglia cardiaca - Pulmonary system - Digestive system
Sympathetic	- Respiratory system - Cardiovascular system - Digestive system

Materials and Methods

We studied 19 patients, 13 females and 6 males, aged 31-72 years, who were admitted to the Gastroenterology Department. These patients were divided in two groups: 14 patients with functional GER disease and, as control group, 5 patients with GER due to hiatal hernia (anatomic alteration). Diagnosis was based on a series of exams including radiography with double contrast (bolus and gas), esophagoscopy with flexible fiberscope, esophageal manometry to study the dynamic and static variations in pressure, and esophageal pH monitoring. All patients had a thorough clinical history, ear, nose and throat (ENT) examination with rigid and flexible endoscopes, anterior rhinomanometry (RRM), skin tests for inhalant and food allergens, radioallergosorbent test (RAST), audiometric exam, paranasal sinus X-rays [18], and non-specific nasal provocation test (NSNPT) with histamine [19-21], using as control the RRM variations and the numbers of sneezes [22-23].

Results

At clinical history, all patients with functional GER disease complained of pharyngeal symptoms, 4 noticed subjective dysphonia, and 2 were worried about their bronchial complaint (Table 2).

Nasal symptoms (e.g. obstruction, sneezes, hydrorrea), mild dysphonia, and cough were referred by the same patients when the physician asked specifically about each anatomical zone, confirming that patients remember only the more annoying symptoms whereas they forget all that they do not consider clinically important.

From a thorough analysis of the objective examination and from the results of the instrumental examinations (Table 3), we found that all patients with functional GER were rhinopathics, even if with different severity and impairments, while this was not true for the small group with GER due to hiatal hernia. In the patients with functional GER pharyngeal involvment was manifested as severe congestion of the posterior wall of the pharynx (with foreign body sensation). In more than half of these patients, chronic Reinke's edema of the vocal cords was evident as was asthmatic involvement of the lower airways. Skin test and RAST for the

Table 2. Symptoms complained of by patients suffering from functional GER or GER caused by hiatal hernia

Symptoms	Functional GER (n = 14)	GER due to hiatal hernia (n = 5)
Nasal	13	0
Obstruction	9	-
Sneezing	7	-
Hydrorrea	2	-
Pharyngeal	14	1
Laryngeal (dysphonia)	7	1
Bronchial	8	0
Cough	5	-
Asthma	3	-

Table 3. Ear, nose and throat (ENT) examination results in patients with functional GER or GER due to hiatal hernia

| | No. patients testing positive | |
Examination	Functional GER (n = 14)	GER due to hiatal hernia (n = 5)
Turbinates, edema	13	1
Turbinates, hypertrophy	7	0
Nasal polyposis	1	0
Pharynx hyperemia/atrophy	12	1
Otoscopy (tympanic retraction)	4	1
Larynx (Reinke's edema)	8	1
Prick test (food, pneumoallergens)	0	0
RAST	0	0
Maxillary sinuses pathology		
Effusion	0	1
Spissitude	9	0
Opacity	5	0
Conductive hearing loss		
Mild	2	1
Moderate	1	0
Severe	0	0

RAST, radioallergosorbent test

common allergens (e.g. pollen, inhalants, mycophages, food) were negative. This was an important parameter because it is not possible to test all substances that potentially may induce an IgE-mediated reaction.

The high percentage of paranasal sinus involvement in these patients is considered normal [18-24]; similar results reported in the literature include:

- 91% among patients with recurrent inflammation due to non-specific hyperreactivity;
- 40.9% in allergic patients (20% in those positive for *Graminacee*, 30% for *Parietaria officinalis*, 76% for *Dermatophagoides pteronissinus*, 4% for others);
- 100% of ASA-intolerant patients [25].

The non-specific nasal provocation test with histamine [26] showed hyperreactivity with sneezes in 9 of 14 patients with functional GER and in 2 of 5 patients with GER due to hiatal hernia. Whereas the RRM results showed unilateral nasal hyperreactivity in 6 of 14 patients with functional GER, 2 did not have any variation. In the group with GER due to hiatal hernia, only 1 patient showed unilateral RRM variation (Table 4, Fig. 1).

Table 4. Resistance score threshold for left and right nasal cavity (*Rleft* and *Rright*, respectively), and numbers of sneezes before and after non-specific nasal provocation test (NSNPT) with histamine

Patient	Pathology	Before		After		No. sneezes
		Rright	Rleft	Rright	Rleft	
1	Hiatal hernia	0.3	0.4	0.9	0.5	3
2	Functional GER	0.27	1.3	1.31	1.73	8
3	Functional GER	0.8	1.3	0.3	1.97	8
4	Functional GER	0.5	0.8	1.1	2.2	5
5	Functional GER	0.09	2.35	0.03	3.49	13
6	Hiatal hernia	0.38	0.6	0.52	0.42	1
7	Hiatal hernia	0.44	0.8	0.36	0.71	0
8	Functional GER	0.19	0.19	4.7	0.75	0
9	Functional GER	0.6	0.5	9.5	1.9	4
10	Hiatal hernia	0.5	0.74	0.37	0.82	0
11	Functional GER	0.78	1.05	2.27	5.0	6
12	Functional GER	0.49	0.84	0.55	3.04	2
13	Functional GER	1.07	0.54	0.81	2.39	3
14	Functional GER	1.89	0.62	3.28	0.85	3

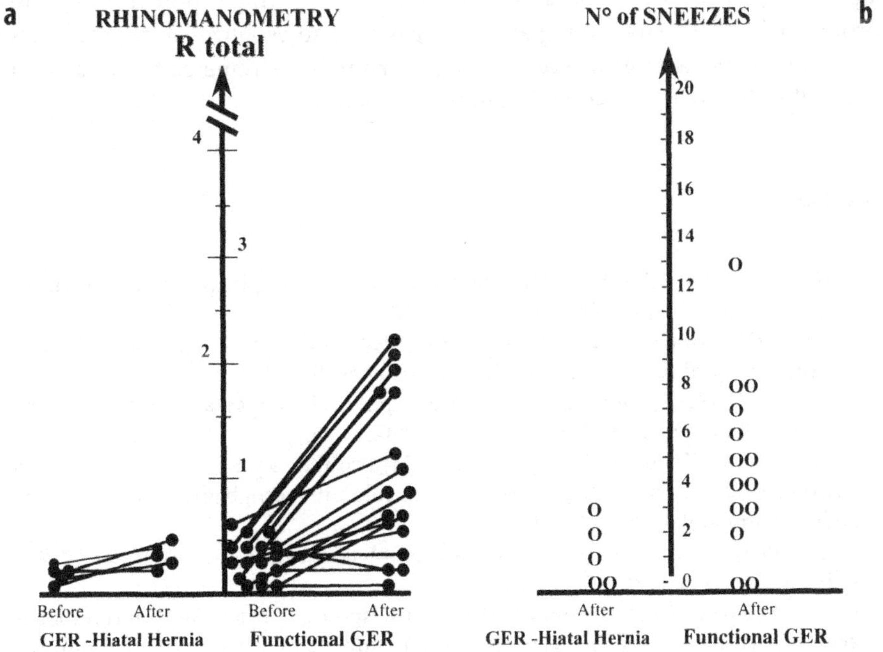

Fig. 1. a Total resistance score threshold for nasal cavities before and after NSNPT with histamine, for patients with functional GER or GER due to hiatal hernia. **b** Number of sneezes after NSNPT with histamine

Discussion

Even if we take into account the small number of the patients under observation, we can not deny the relevance of the data reported in this study, even though they need further confirmation. The existence of two pathological forms of GER, one primary and one secondary, is evident. The latter is always preceded by upper airways pathology. The non-specific hyperreactivity of the upper aerodigestive tract and the following release of the lower esophageal sphincter (introduction of reflux) could represent pathological pictures linked to chronic environmental stimulation. In particular, the neurogenic component of inflammation due to hyperreactivity could cause a greater upregulation of irritant receptors with the consequent involvement of vagal fibers at the soft palate and pharynx, and the possible transfer of stimuli to the esophageal sphincter.

Therefore, Mansfield and Stein's theory [16], which hypothesizes a pathology mediated by the vagus nerve appears to be valid. So does our hypothesis that the stimulus which excites the vagus nerve may be present in food (or in additives, colorants, and antibiotics) and may arrive by nasal-oral inspiration. These irritants stimulate the vagal nerve endings in the soft palate, and in the posterior walls of the pharynx and larynx. The chronicity of the problem could cause release of the smooth musculature of the esophageal sphincter, giving rise to a pathology whose symptomatology could let the starting problem pass on to a secondary level. The damaging action of gastric and esophageal juice refluxes on the muscarinic laryngeal receptors may permit, in extreme cases, inhalation of the acid reflux without coughing in these patients.

References

1. Frank M, Komisar A (1993) Ambulatory pH monitoring in the management of reflux. Ann Otol Rhinol Laryngol 102:243-246
2. Burton DM, Pransky SM, Katz RM (1992) Pediatric airways manifestations of gastroesophageal reflux. Ann Otol Rhinol Laryngol 101:742-749
3. Kennedy JH (1962) "Silent" gastroesophageal reflux. An important but little known cause of pulmonary complications. Dis Chest 42:42-45
4. Orenstein SR, Kocoshis SA, Orenstein DM, Proujansky R (1987) Stridor and gastroesophageal reflux: diagnostic use of intraluminal esophageal acid perfusion. Pediatr Pulmonol 3:420-424
5. Orenstein SR, Orenstein DM (1988) Gastroesophageal reflux and respiratory disease in children. J Pediatr 112:847-858
6. Davis RS, Larsen GL, Grunstein MM (1983) Respiratory response to intraesophageal acid infusion in asthmatic children during sleep. J Allergy Clin Immunol 72:393-398
7. Herve P, Denjean A, Jian R, Simonneau G, Duroux P (1986) Intraesophageal perfusion of acid increases the bronchomotor response to metacholine and to isocapnic hyperventilation in asthmatic patients. Am Rev Respir Dis 134:986-989

8. Toohill RJ, Mushtag E, Lehman RH (1990) Otolaryngologic manifestations of gastroesophageal reflux. In: Sacristan T, Alvarez-Vicent JJ, Bartual J, Antoli-Candela F, Rubio L (eds) Proceedings of the 24th World Congress of Otorhinolaryngology Head and Neck Surgery. Kugler and Ghedini, Amsterdam, pp 3005-3009

9. Koufman JA (1991) The otolaryngologic manifestations of gastroesophageal reflux disease (GERD). Laryngoscope 101(4 Pt 2 Suppl 53):1-78

10. Bain WM, Harrington JW, Thomas LE, Schefer SD (1983) Head and neck manifestations of gastroesophageal reflux. Laryngoscope 93:175-179

11. Gumpert L, Kalach N, Dupont C, Contencin P (1998) Hoarseness and gastroesophageal reflux. J Otol Laryngol 112:49-54

12. Richtsmeier WJ, Styczynski P, Johns ME (1987) Selective histamine-mediated immunosuppresion in laryngeal cancer. Ann Otol Rhinol Laryngol 96:569-572

13. Jindal JR, Milbrath M, Shaker R, Hogan WJ, Toohill RJ (1994) Gastroesophageal reflux disease as likely cause of "idiopathic" subglottic stenosis. Ann Otol Rhinol Laryngol 103:186-191

14. Zeitels SM, Hillman RE, Bunting GW, Vaughin T (1997) Reinke's edema: phonatory mechanisms and management strategies. Ann Otol Rhinol Laryngol 106:533-543

15. Bauman NM, Sandler AD, Smith RJH (1996) Respiratory manifestations of gastroesophageal reflux disease in pediatric patients. Ann Otol Rhinol Laryngol 105:23-32

16. Mansfield LE, Stein MR (1978) Gastroesophageal reflux and asthma: a possible reflex mechanism. Ann Allergy 41:224-226

17. Rival R, Wong R, Mendelsohn M, Rosgen S, Freeman J (1995) Role of gastroesophageal reflux disease in patients with cervical symptoms. Otolaryngol Head Neck Surg 113:364-369

18. Filiaci F, Zambetti (1988) Rhinitis. Perspectives in ENT-Immunology 2:36-47

19. Corrado OJ, Gould CA, Kassad JY (1986) Nasal response of rhinitic and non-rhinitic subjects to histamine and methacoline. Thorax 41:863-868

20. Filiaci F, Zambetti G (1983) Aspecific nasal reactivity in allergic and nonallergic subjets. Rhinology 21:329-334

21. Filiaci F, Zambetti G, Lo Vecchio A, Romeo R (1996) The behaviour of nonspecific nasal provocation tests in subjects with allergic rhinitis and not, in and out of crisis: a longitudinal study. Allergol Immunopathol 24:98-102

22. Filiaci F, Zambetti G, Luce M (1994) Local therapy with capsaicin in vasomotor rhinopathy. Allergol Immunopathol 22:264-268

23. Filiaci F, Zambetti G, Ciofalo A (1996) Local treatment with capsaicin in patients affected by nonspecific nasal hyperreactivity: a longitudinal study. Allergologie vereinigt mit Allergie und Immunologie 19:40

24. Crifò S, Filiaci F (1974) House-dust mite nasal allergies. Rhinology 12:79-84

25. Shaker R, Millbrath M, Ren J, Toohill R, Hogan WJ, Li Q, Hoffman CL (1995) Esophagopharyngeal distribution of refluxed gastric acid in patients with reflux laryngitis. Gastroenterology 109:1575-1582

26. Zambetti G, Moresi M, Filiaci F (1998) Nonspecific nasal provocation test with histamine: analysis of the dose/response curve. Preliminary results. Am J Rhinol (in press)

Bronchial Asthma and GER

L. ALLEGRA

Introduction

In 1935, Winkelstein proposed a new pathological entity called peptic esophagitis [1]. Several years later the term reflux esophagitis was introduced to indicate the pathophysiological mechanism underlying the disease [2]. It was later demonstrated that gastroesophageal reflux (GER) may occur even in the absence of esophagitis, and the more comprehensive term gastroesophageal reflux disease (GERD) was introduced, to include disturbances and disease processes due to GERD that involve other organs besides the esophagus. Specific attention has been drawn to diseases of the respiratory tract: association with asthma (although hypothesized by Sir W. Osler a long time ago [3] and sporadically mentioned thereafter [4, 5]) and chronic bronchitis was described in the late 1970s [6-8] with a progressively increasing interest [9-19], whereas an association between reflux and idiopathic pulmonary fibrosis (IPF) was suggested in the 1960s [20] and confirmed successively [21-25]. Other respiratory disturbances such as persistent chronic cough [26-29] and nocturnal asphyxia in children [30] were reported later than asthma and IPF. Further associations, although not supported scientifically have been suspected (e.s. bronchiectasis, hemoptysis). Proof has been given regarding the relationship between GER and hoarseness [31] or far more severe upper airway diseases [32, 33] such as acute or chronic laryngitis [34-38], laryngeal ulcers [39] and even glottic carcinoma [40, 41].

Among respiratory diseases associated with GER, asthma is the most extensively studied and has gathered the most convincing data. Asthma occurs in patients with hyperresponsive airways that manifest bronchoconstriction in response to a variety of stimuli. The disease is often etiologically multifactorial. GER is undoubtfully a triggering mechanism, but it may also act as a causal factor in asthma. Bronchial epithelium plays a pivotal role in asthma: it is highly susceptible to pH variations along its surface (as may occur during microaspiration of gastric material), to vagus-mediated reflexes as is the case of reflux-induced bronchoconstrictor

Institute of Respiratory Diseases, University of Milan, IRCCS Ospedale Maggiore, Milan, Italy

reflexes, and perhaps to other GER-induced mechanisms of disturbance (see further on: The GER-Asthma Hypothesis: Pathogenesis of GER-correlated Asthma).

Definition of GER

Gastroesophageal reflux (GER) is today a well-defined, independent pathological entity, often confused with other digestive diseases and therefore still underestimated and underrated in its true epidemiological impact. For over two decades, epidemiological studies from various countries have demonstrated that gastroesophageal reflux is, in absolute terms, one of the most common gastrointestinal disturbances. Moreover, recent studies have shown that GER may play a role in upper and lower respiratory tract diseases.

GER may be defined as a *dysfunction of the lower esophagus which causes abnormal passage of gastric contents into the esophagus*. It should be noted that mild GER occurring after a meal must be considered physiological, particularly during early infancy or pregnancy.

Elements of Anatomy of the Lower Esophagus

The lower esophagus crosses the diaphragm at the esophageal hiatus and therefore includes an abdominal tract (Fig. 1). The lower esophageal portion is a physiological sphincter, lacking a true anatomical identity. Proceeding caudally a slightly dilated segment is observed: the epiphrenic ampulla, then the vestibule, and lastly the gastroesophageal junction or anatomical cardias.

From a functional standpoint, the vestibule coincides with the lower esophageal sphincter (LES) (Fig. 2).

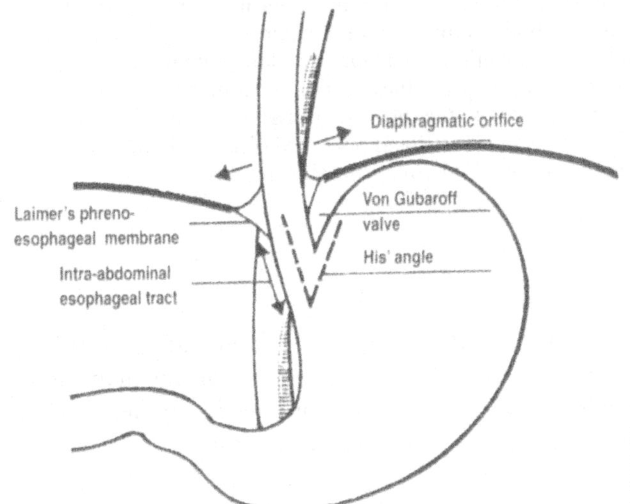

Fig. 1. The gastroesophageal junction: an anatomical antireflux barrier. (From [42] with permission, modified)

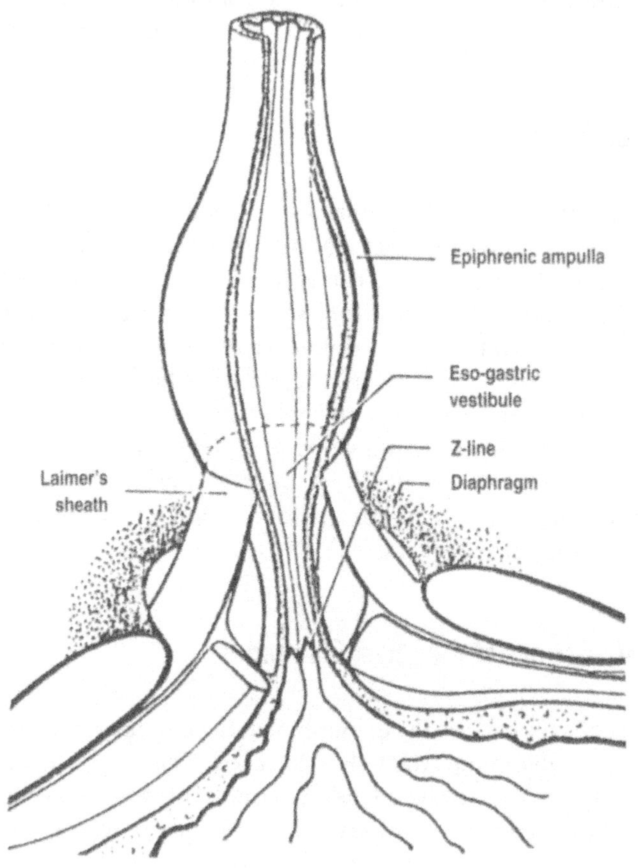

Fig. 2. Comparison between anatomical radio-endoscopic and manometric aspects of the lower esophagus. When contracted (*dotted line*), the gastroesophageal vestibule coincides with an area of endoluminal occlusion, both from radiographic and endoscopic points of view. Radiographically, the cephalad accumulation of barium forms the epiphrenic ampulla. When dilated, particularly under endoscopic inflation, the vestibular tract appears marked by two ring-like zones, corresponding to the insertion of Laimer's sheath. In a case of hiatal hernia, endoscopic inflation determines the appearance of a third ring, corresponding to the diaphragmatic hiatus. (From [42] with permission, modified)

Pathogenesis of GER

The fundamental pathogenic factor in GER is the competence of the lower esophageal sphincter (LES). Resting basal LES tone is less important than the sphincter's capacity to dilate when physiologically appropriate, i.e. immediately after swallowing. In particular, pathogenic factors can be identified as:

- Antireflux barrier efficacy
- Gastric content volume
- Esophageal clearing efficacy
- Damaging properties of the refluxing material
- Resistance to damage and regenerative capacity of the esophageal structure.

When and why reflux becomes symptomatic has not been completely clarified yet. It is likely that the complex interactions which regulate LES tone, i.e. peristalsis and release, are altered. Among leading abnormalities, a key role is probably played by:
- Fall in LES resting pressure to < 10 mm Hg
- Decrease in LES adaptive response to increases in intra-abdominal pressure
- Defective post-prandial gastrin release
- Hyperlipidic diet
- Use of beta-2-agonists, theophylline, calcium channel blockers, benzodiazepines, etc.

The role of *hiatal hernia* needs to be briefly discussed. Some authors argue that the role of hiatal hernia in GER should be reduced to that of a simple reflux cofactor [12]. It has been shown that during esophageal clearing, small quantities of acidic material are trapped within the hernial sack and hence flow back into the esophagus when the sphincter dilates during subsequent swallowing: repeated episodes of hiatal hernia reflux explain the prolonged overall esophageal clearing time observed in patients with hernia.

However, many Authors [4, 24, 43, 44] have observed that hiatal hernia may be demonstrated in a high percentage of subjects with asthma and other lung diseases, particularly when bronchial symptoms appear or worsen late in life and also when the subject is not necessarily free from other potential causes of asthma (asthma can be monofactorial, for example due to GER only, but also multifactorial with causes of asthma other than GER, allergies included).

The GER-Asthma Hypothesis: Pathogenesis of GER-correlated Asthma

The association between GER and respiratory disease is now well known. Until not long ago, it was thought that GER could determine respiratory disorders by aspiration of gastric material into the airways. We must distinguish between macroaspiration [43-45] (or "flooding") of the tracheobronchial tree (which leads to clinical entities such as aspiration pneumonitis, lung abscess, bronchiectasis) and microaspiration [9], a mechanism specially invoked for GER-induced asthma [46, 47]. Recently, studies have shown the importance of vagus-mediated reflex mechanisms: bronchoconstriction, laryngeal spasm, central apnea and reflex bradycardia [48, 49].

The common occurrence of GER in patients with asthma has been demonstrated in various recent studies. This phenomenon has been observed in all types of bronchial asthma, although prevalently in severe chronic asthma, in adult-onset asthma, in asthma associated with nasal polyposis, in perimenstrual or perimenopausal asthma or in asthma occurring during pregnancy. Numerous complications result from this association; the most interesting concern the mechanisms causing the onset or worsening of asthma symptoms. We feel there are several possible explanations for this, the first three being shared by the majority of authors (Table 1):

a) Microaspiration of refluxing material, sometimes with aerosol generation (gastric secretions, food, sometimes biliary material) beyond the epiglottis which results in inflammation and airway obstruction [50-54].

b) Broncho-esophageal vagal reflexes triggered by esophageal acidification, known as "reflux-induced reflex"; aerosolized refluxing material may stimulate acid sensitive receptors present on the pharyngeal portion of the esophagus and cause bronchoconstriction [8, 55-58].

c) GER-induced heightening of bronchial hyperreactivity, postulated through the exalted level of non-specific airway responsiveness to challenges such as methacholine, histamine, or isocapnic hyperventilation [59, 60].

d) A fourth hypothesis we can propose [61], perhaps less frequent, but still present at least as a cofactor and often identified by the radiologists, is that in subjects with reversible (as in asthma) or non-reversible (as in emphysema) hyperinflation of airspaces, there may be a flattening of the diaphragm, modifying the His' angle from acute to obtuse and determining traction on the LES and loss of its competence with the consequent vicious circle hyperinflation-reflux-asthma (Fig. 3).

e) The last, purely hypothetical, possibilities we can propose (unpublished observations) consist of the onset of allergic phenomena with reaginic response to alimentary allergens, due to "increased esophageal permeability" in the refluent patients, or to patients' sensitization to food allergens reaching the lungs and being absorbed.

Table 1. Possible mechanisms causing GER-induced asthmatic symptoms

Microaspiration of gastric refluxing material
Vagally mediated reflux-induced reflex
Reflux-induced heightening of bronchial responsiveness
Vicious circle: hyperinflation-reflux-asthma
Increased esophageal permeability to alimentary allergens
Alimentary allergens refluent into the airways

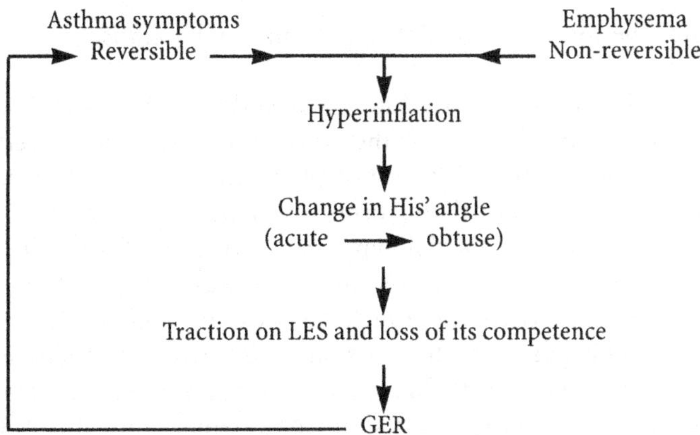

Fig. 3. Hypothesis of vicious circle

The relationship between asthma and GER may become clinically apparent in two ways, each distinct from an etiological and physiological standpoint: (a) reflux-associated onset of asthma or (b) reflux which appears during the evolution of clinically present asthma.

The clinical characteristics of reflux-associated asthma allow the identification of a unique syndrome; from the onset, symptoms are severe and invalidating. There is an initial nocturnal prevalence due to postural factors (supine position) which favour reflux activity. Exacerbations are invariably anticipated by severe tracheitis with cough bouts, often occurring a long time before dyspnea appears. Clinical characteristics are also often very distinctive and immediately evocative. Severe, easily identifiable and poorly tolerated symptoms are almost always involved.

Significantly, a detailed past history may reveal a precise time association between respiratory and digestive symptoms, the former often becoming evident years after the onset of the latter. It has been shown [4, 62] that between 16% and 70% of adult patients with bronchial asthma present symptoms due to gastroesophageal reflux, as demonstrated by the use of esophageal radiograms, endoscopy, esophageal pH recordings and manometry [15]. Furthermore Ducoloné et al. [12] monitored esophageal pH after meals, showing GER in the large majority of chronic bronchitic patients, and suggested that in such patients reflux may be prolonged in time, whereas in asthma patients reflux episodes are more frequent but short-lasting. In patients with chronic obstructive pulmonary disease, Crausaz and Favez [13] observed the existence of GER in 84% of cases, and pulmonary microaspiration in 75% of cases. During the study period, traces of vegetable fibers were found in sputum samples from both patients and control group subjects. This finding was in contrast with scintiscan observations. However, these authors believe aspiration of saliva into the upper airways (up to the trachea) to be a physiological event, whereas "pathological" aspiration of gastric content into the lower airways in asthmatic patients justifies the increased incidence of "abnormal" scintiscan findings in these patients.

Vagus-mediated bronchoconstriction was first demonstrated by Mansfield and Stein [8]. The stimulus is given by the presence of acidic gastric secretions in the lower esophagus. The reflex is not physiological, since it cannot be evoked in healthy subjects: pre-existing bronchial hyperresponsiveness is a necessary requirement. In turn, bronchial hyperreactivity in itself is insufficient: in some asthma patients reflux does not cause any worsening of the disease. Moreover, there are cases where no bronchoconstriction occurs after acidification of the lower esophagus (Bernstein test) and cases where antireflux therapy is ineffective in asthma patients. Reflux is only found in some patients, presumably in the presence of vagal hyperexcitability or a strong cholinergically mediated hypersensitivity. Once reflux has been identified, the clinical problem is the precise definition of its role in terms of respiratory therapy. The discriminative role of the Bernstein test has recently been questioned and lessened by some authors. The low percentage of Bernstein-positive subjects among asthma patients with GER (< 10% in our series) is obviously due to the fact that the pathogenetic modality indicated as reflux-induced reflex is much less frequent than the microaspirative modality. That both these mechanisms can occur in mammals has been demonstrated in animal models by us, and is discussed elsewhere in this volume [63].

One can presume reflux to play a role in the pathogenesis of bronchial asthma even in the absence of microaspiration which is, however, the most frequent case in our series: microaspiration has been proven by pulmonary scintiscan positivity 12 hours after the ingestion of a radioactive Tc-labeled drink in 63% of patients with GER-correlated asthma. It is difficult to imagine the pathogenetic mechanism in the remaining cases of GER-correlated or GER-induced asthma or when diagnosis is confirmed by a successful ex juvantibus gastric therapy where the Bernstein test is negative and microaspiration is not demonstrated. Either inconsistency of methods or other possible pathogenetic mechanisms may be claimed. In this setting, lung function testing plays an important role in recording the presence of bronchoconstriction coinciding with reflux episodes. The following tests are of use: spirometry, transcutaneous determination of pO_2 and pCO_2, inductive plethysmography, and recording airflow at the mouth and pressures in the esophagus and above the glottis. A reliable method for determining the correlation between episodes of GER and variations in lung function is the simultaneous monitoring of esophageal pH and intrathoracic pulmonary resistance. Using this technique in selected asthma patients with severe reflux-induced disease and endoscopically proven esophagitis, a 4-5 fold increase in pulmonary resistance compared to baseline values immediately before the reflux episode was recorded [64]. After medical antireflux treatment, these same patients showed a significant reduction in the episodes of nocturnal bronchoconstriction together with the elimination of the morning fall in peak expiratory flow. This shows that under specific circumstances GER may act as a bronchoconstrictive stimulus.

Therefore, GER plays a relevant and decisive role in the complex pathogenic mechanisms of bronchial asthma. In a certain number of cases it may be considered a causal factor for asthma [65]. It is nonetheless advisable to investigate its presence and characteristics even in cases of asthma where the etiological agents are certain (e.g. cases where a bronchoconstrictive response to allergens has been demonstrated). It must not be forgotten that asthma is often multifactorial and it may not be appropriate to terminate investigations once a single factor has been identified.

Partial, prevalent or exclusive involvement of GER should be considered in the presence of: (a) unexplained long-lasting cough in subjects who have no bronchial hyperresponsiveness; (b) adult or senile-onset asthma; (c) hiatal hernia or gastric disease in asthmatic patients; (d) perimenopausal/premenstrual asthma symptoms or asthma episodes during the first three months of pregnancy (estrogen and hormone bursts cause esophageal dilation); (e) laryngitis, rhinosinusitis, nasal polyps, otitis of the middle ear, or tear duct disturbances in association with asthma; (f) intolerance to antiasthmatic drugs such as theophylline preparations, strong doses of beta-2-agonists, all which act not only as bronchodilators but also as esophageal dilators; (g) intolerance to systemic steroids and non-steroid anti-inflammatory drugs (NSAID) which cause gastritis and increase gastric acid production, aumenting the damaging effects in case of reflux; (h) gallbladder diseases or surgical removal in the patient's history with consequent alkaline reflux, relatively infrequent in patients with GER-induced asthma (unfortunately more difficult to demonstrate now that the esophageal pH probe in general is calibrated only for acid pH, and unfortunately also difficult to cure because of the obvious inefficiency of the antiacid therapy. A mixed acid and alkaline reflux is also possible.

The Detrimental Activity of GER on Respiratory Health: From Suspicion to Ascertainment

The possible pulmonary manifestations and the severity of the effects of GER may vary considerably [8, 66]. GER may act as the main cause of respiratory disease, but these may in turn contribute to the onset or worsening of GER, thus creating in many cases a vicious circle [15, 16]. A clinical description of the pulmonary consequences of gastric fluid inhalation was first given by Allison in 1946 [2]. The degree of damage is associated with the quantity of inhaled liquid, its pH, and presence of food microparticles.

Multiple microaspiration of gastric contents into the lower airway induces damage to the respiratory bronchioles and to the alveolar structures with an initial inflammatory response which can be followed by pulmonary fibrosis. Lung damage can be divided into three broad categories:
- Chemical bronchiolitis with damage to the capillary-alveolar membrane and reduced surfactant production, leading to microatelectasis, necrotic destruction of the alveolar epithelial and/or endothelial cells and proliferation of type II pneumocytes.

- Inflammatory response to the presence of food microparticles in the airways, with polymorphous cellular infiltration of plasmocytes and large numbers of neutrophils and eosinophils into the intralveolar septa.
- Infection which may occur when the inhaled fluid pH is above 2.5; in these conditions the fluid often harbors anerobic bacteria from the oropharynx [67] and superinfection with aerobic gram-negative bacteria and/or staphylococci may occur [68]. Demonstration of gastric content aspiration into the airways is complex (detection of lipid- or lactose-laden macrophages in tracheobronchial specimens or positive scintiscan following, hours later or after overnight, radioisotopic-labelled material ingestion), and is limited by false-positive and false-negative results.

GER may be suspected in patients with depressed conscience, altered neurophysiological co-ordination mechanisms with suffocation or coughing during meals, or abnormal chest X-ray findings. Evening gastroesophageal scintigraphy followed by pulmonary scintiscan in the morning may confirm clinical suspicions. A controlled study by Mays et al. [24] found that 73% of patients with idiopathic pulmonary fibrosis (IPF) in the absence of immunological disorders had a hiatal hernia and 44% presented GER, whereas in control subjects hernia and GER were present in 19% and 5% of cases, respectively. In an earlier study, Pearson and Wilson [21] monitored a vast population for GER symptoms and noticed the presence of clinical and radiological signs of IPF in 6% of the patients. Quite recently, the high prevalence of the association GER-IPF has been not only confirmed but also observed in a high percentage of IPF patients who do not suffer any typical clinical symptom of GER [25].

GER with aspiration has been demonstrated in some cases of pneumonia and pulmonary abscesses. Repeated aspiration episodes over time may cause recurrent or granulomatous pneumonia and chronic bronchitis. Berquist et al. [43] observed digestive symptoms indicating the presence of GER in 18% of children with recurrent pneumonia, whereas in 43% the presence of GER was demonstrated by esophageal manometry and pH monitoring. In these small patients chest X-ray showed lung infiltrates primarily in the middle and lower right lobes or the lingula. Patients presenting aspiration who underwent surgical fundoplication presented no relapse at a 15-month follow-up [22, 23].

A further condition associated with GER is laryngeal spasm. It typically arises in unweaned children; in severe cases it can cause apnea and sudden death [69, 70]. Laryngeal stridor represents an incomplete form of reflex laryngeal spasm; this condition must not be confused with laryngomalacia. Patients present a dry unresponsive cough, thoracic constriction, and dyspnea. The greater degree of severity in unweaned children is due to anatomical factors, such as limited upper airway cross-sectional area and neurological limitations. The symptoms of reflex laryngeal spasm are fairly typical: the child is awake and often presents repeated episodes of regurgitation. Approximately one hour after a meal, while sitting or in supine position, the child has an apnea crisis, with eyes wide open in a fixed stare. Opisthotonus, pallor, and cyanosis are usually present. Medical antireflux therapy, or occasionally surgery, are capable of reverting respiratory symptoms. The pathogenetic mechanisms are as yet unknown; the search for the neurological pathways and the receptors involved has so far been inconclusive.

Cough as a symptom is often useful in distinguishing between different diseases of the respiratory tract. It is generally possible to reach a diagnosis on the basis of the clinical characteristics of different forms of cough. This is not always so, and unexplained cough is sometimes referred to as "cough of unknown origin". Irwin et al. [71] demonstrated that 10% of persistent, chronic cough cases were due to GER. In these patients, detailed past history investigations revealed the presence of digestive symptoms indicating GER, 24-hour esophageal pH monitoring showed reflux episodes with pH < 4 lasting > 5 min, and endoscopy revealed signs of esophagitis. The same group of authors later demonstrated [27, 28] that in patients with chronic cough and history indicating previous reflux episodes, GER was the predominant cause of coughing, which improved considerably or completely disappeared following medical anti-reflux therapy. Reversal of cough as a symptom is a long process because medical therapy decreases, but does not completely eliminate, reflux episodes. This slow disappearance of cough is associated with slow healing of the lower esophageal mucosa which is still exposed to the action of low pH reflux, although qualitatively and quantitatively less intense.

Our Overall Experience on the GER-Asthma Hypothesis

Within the limits of the pathologic "respiratory" patient histories, particular attention has to be paid in individualizing the signals and the suggestive symptoms of gastroesophageal reflux disease. The particular pathologic definition has assumed in recent years a heterogeneous characteristic, including not only the acid reflux effects on the esophageal mucosa but also those on the larynx and on pulmonary symptoms. The pulmonary manifestations during the course of GERD can be quite diverse, ranging from a dry chronic cough to recurrent aspiration pneumonia. Among those already stated above, particular importance must be given to asthma: if asthma can worsen the already existent reflux, more frequent observations suggest that the same reflux could be a strong bronchoconstrictive stimulus.

The incidence of gastroesophageal reflux in asthma patients is certainly superior to that which is found in the general population. The importance of GERD during infancy must be noted. Andze et al. [72], for example, in 500 children with asthma, found that over 60% had GERD and of those, 41% had "severe" reflux.

Considering adult patients alone, we have systematically recorded, over 15 years, GER symptoms in asthma patients (1164 cases out of 2044 consecutively investigated asthma patients, 57%): all patients came to our center spontaneously, i.e. independently of referral centers. GER acted as a clinically relevant cofactor in 47% (657/1381) of patients with extrinsic asthma: in these patients addition of GER medical therapy alone was fundamental in improving symptom scores or eliminating symptoms. In 32% of our patients, no clinically evident form of allergy was detected: in 76% (507/663) of these "nonallergic" patients we found evidence of GER, and both digestive and respiratory symptoms were corrected by the introduction of dietary restrictions, by lifting the upper part of the patient's bed, and by treatment with alginate and omeprazole (less frequently alginate and ranidine) plus cisapride. Even more significant is the number of cases of clinically relevant GER in nonallergic subjects with adult-onset asthma (> 45 years of age): in this subgroup of patients (n = 248), the presence of GER was demonstrated in 199 cases (80%), with clinical improvement after medical antireflux therapy. In two-thirds of these patients (132/199, 61%), a hiatal hernia was identified (all X-rays viewed by the same radiologist), and in 15/16 (94%) chronic asthma subjects with clear-cut emphysema but no detectable hernia, a modification of the His' angle (from acute to obtuse) was observed (see Figs. 1 and 3).

Most epidemiological data on the prevalence of GER in asthma indicate rates between 34% and 89%, as opposed to a 5%-19% rate in control groups (non-asthmatic subjects). The differences recorded, in diverse study populations, explain the apparently widely differing prevalence rates found in different case series. Due to the lack of precise epidemiological studies carried out on the general population (for example, as assessed by electoral lists), the percentage most often expresses the reflexed patient stratification based on age, sex, presence of allergy, coexistence of hiatal hernia, non-reversible lung hyperinflation (emphysema), etc. In other words, there are numerous variables that may change according to the study population and the center in which the study is carried out. Our overmentioned data, for example, refer exclusively to an outpatient, private, nonpediatric pneumological center (not an "asthma-center") known for its studies on intrinsic asthma, so that a strong qualitative difference between our cases and those which can be assessed by a pediatric or allergologic center or by a center with a primary vocation to asthma can be considered normal.

Patient Examination

History

Meticulous attention must be given to gathering a detailed history for all asthmatic patients, particularly when determining: (a) presence of GER; (b) hypothetical causes determining GER; and (c) the clinical relevance of GER in determining or contributing to symptoms of bronchoconstriction. The reason for paying particular attention to previous history information lies in the fact that the patient is rarely aware of a cause-effect relationship between respiratory symptoms and esophageal disease. The patient is often surprised, and sometimes annoyed, that a lung specialist consulted for a respiratory ailment shifts attention to the digestive system, applying the same detailed investigation used for respiratory system. The patient therefore initially responds superficially or reluctantly until it slowly becomes apparent that the questions asked reflect the true nature of the symptoms experienced. At this point the patient's attention and curiosity has been captured by this intriguing new hypothesis regarding "difficult" asthma symptoms that had often been considered indomitable in previous consultations.

At this point, enquiries should point to dietary habits and medication use, which often reveal intolerance or gastric symptoms (heartburn or pyrosis) due to ingestion of alcohol, tea, coffee, chocolate, citrus fruits, soup, lipid-rich meals, tomatoes, mint, onion, garlic, spices, liquorice, soft drinks, theophylline, beta-2-agonists, female hormones, or oral steroids.

Sleep habits have then to be investigated: sleepiness immediately after a meal, preferred body position, if sleeping with more than one pillow or elevated head-rest is preferred, if nocturnal symptoms are present, and if sleeping on one side limits or eliminates disturbing awakenings.

Questions must be asked regarding selected times of the day at which bronchoconstrictive events appear (evening, after a meal, or at night), coexistence of hoarseness on awakening, snoring, drooling, foreign body sensation in the throat, or food regurgitation.

The patient must be helped to remember the onset of the digestive complaint, observing possible associations with the onset (or worsening) of asthma symptoms. It will therefore be possible to detect the high frequency of nonallergic, adult-or senile-onset, reflux-associated asthma. These patients are often aware of the presence of a hiatal hernia but have never suspected a possible association between asthma and reflux disease.

In females, the chronological association between asthma and menstrual cycle (asthma in puberty, asthma during menstrual cycle) or menopause must be investigated. Female hormones do not directly influence asthma, but bursts of both estrogens and progesterone are recognized as factors influencing LES competence. Reflux occurring during the first 3 months of pregnancy may be associated with asthma via the above-reported mechanisms. Reflux-induced asthma during the last three months of pregnancy is more likely to be due to mechanical factors linked to an increase in abdominal pressure.

Asthmogenic GER May Be a Reality When:

- Asthma symptoms recur in the perimenstrual or perimenopausal period
- Asthma symptoms recur in the first trimester of pregnancy
- Asthma symptoms recur in the third trimester of pregnancy
- First onset of asthma in adult/senile age
- History of dyspepsia, gastritis, ulcer, *Helicobacter pylory* infection, hiatal hernia, epigastric pain or spontaneous use of antacids in asthmatics
- History of gallbladder disease or cholecystectomy (alkaline or mixed reflux)
- Asthma symptoms in patients with altered swallowing mechanisms, with suffocation or coughing during meals.

Classic GER Symptoms Are:

- Regurgitation
- Heartburn
- Dysphagia
- Odynophagia
- Chest pain.

Thinking to GER is not pleonastic in the following cases:
- Hoarseness that is recurrent or frequent, specially when awakening
- Preferential lateral decubitus during night
- Asthmatic symptoms impaired by the use of theophyllines, NSAID, non-inhaled steroids, noninhaled beta-2-adrenergics, noninhaled antimuscarinic drugs
- Asthmatic symptoms impaired by fast diet, tomatoes, citrus fruits, kiwis, bananas, sugar, onion, garlic, fenel, peas, beans, meat soup, tea, coffee, chocolate, sparkling drinks, alcoholic drinks, mint, liquorice
- Persistent unexplained cough, specially at night
- Sialorrhea
- Acid, bitter, salty or "metallic" saliva
- Bronchial hypersecretion
- Nasal polyposis, chronic rhinosinusitis with or without otitis media, with or without lacrimal channel disturbances
- Erosion of dental enamel
- "Globus" and/or sensation of laryngotracheal compression perceived in correspondence of UES (upper esophageal sphincter)
- Swallowing difficulties
- Prolonged hiccup duration or rebel hiccups
- Frequent voice clearing
- Frequent nightly awakenings with wheezing, breathlessness, regurgitation, hyperventilation need, or sweating
- Wheezing or dyspnea facilitated by postprandial sleep or change from ortho- to clinostatic position
- Preference for semiorthopnoic position or use of more than one pillow during sleep
- Acid laryngitis
- Posterior chronic laryngitis
- Selective pain at the subxiphoideal digital pressure
- Wheezing appearance or enhancement during maneuvers which increase intra-dominal pressure (weight lifting, difficult defecation, isometric gymnastics, gymnastics for the strengthening of abdominal muscles, bending over)
- Emotions or rage
- Apnea, laryngospasm, respiratory arrest, sudden infant death syndrome.

GER Diagnostic Procedures

Diagnostic procedures for GER include different investigative techniques through which it is possible to identify the presence, severity, and number of reflux episodes in 24 hours, the causes which determine GER, and the correlation with asthma symptoms [73]. Some of these methods have a purely historical value, whereas others are still in use and yield optimal results. By following an accurate diagnostic pathway it is possible to limit procedures to cases where it is truly needed. Some of the procedures in use to ascertain the presence of GER are invasive and bothersome for patients, and should therefore be limited to situations where GER is strongly suspected [74]. No test, in general, will individually ensure the diagnosis of GER (Table 2).

Table 2. Diagnostic tests for the detection of GER

Roentgenography
Esophageal manometry
Esophageal pH monitoring
Esophageal scintigraphy followed by pulmonary scintiscan
Ultrasonography
Esophageal endoscopy
Bernstein test
Ex-juvantibus test

Instrumental procedures for the diagnosis of GER can be divided into three groups:

1. *Tests which demonstrate that reflux is potentially present:*
a) Barium contrast X-ray examination of the esophagus and stomach (possibly demonstrating the presence of a hiatal hernia).
b) Esophageal manometry (demonstrating the existence of pressure conditions which favor reflux).

2. *Tests which demonstrate actual reflux:*
a) Barium contrast X-ray examination of the esophagus and stomach (reflux of contrast medium is sometimes directly visible during the course of the radiographic examination).
b) Esophageal pH monitoring. (From a respiratory point of view, stricter standards such as pH < 3 should be used. It must furthermore be considered that from the pneumologist's point of view reflux episodes lasting even a few seconds are sufficient to induce reflux-induced reflex, whereas gastroenterologists require reflux episodes > 5 min, being mainly interested in determining reflux-induced anatomical esophageal damage).
c) Evening esophageal scintigraphy followed by a pulmonary scintiscan the morning after (detects the arrival of radioisotopes in the lung due to reflux and microaspiration, but may also determine the presence of altered esophageal motility requiring the addition of prokinetics to GER treatment).
d) Ultrasonography.

3. *Tests which give information on the reflux effects:*
a) Esophageal endoscopy with biopsy specimens for cytologic and histologic analysis.
b) The Bernstein test (instillation of 0.1 N HCl into the esophagus not only induces pain and heartburn but also may determine bronchoconstriction).
c) Ex-juvantibus effects of a purely antireflux treatment, alone or added to the previous (e.g. anti-asthmatic) therapy.

Radiographic barium contrast examination is usually the first step taken in the presence of symptoms indicating GER [75]. However, although important for any evaluation of suspected GERD associated with airway disease, barium contrast is scarcely reliable due to difficulties in detecting moderate reflux and to the high number of false-negative results [76]. This technique gives no indication of reflux severity or nocturnal episodes, and does not distinguish between physiological and pathological reflux activity. On the other hand, it allows the identification of any anatomical alteration, such as hiatal hernia. The test requires a certain degree of patient collaboration and particular expertise on the part of the radiologist (particularly if done with air contrast) who must induce the patient to perform adequate maneuvers.

Esophageal manometry is mandatory for measuring upper esophageal sphincter, main body of the esophagus, and LES pressures. This technique demonstrates LES incompetence or hypotonia. Manometry is particularly useful in patients with atypical symptoms (chest pain with vomiting, regurgitation at night only, asthma symptoms) and in patients with typical symptoms who are unresponsive to medical therapy. It allows the recording of intraluminal pressures, generated by phasic contraction of the gastrointestinal wall, giving information on upper and lower esophageal sphincter pressures, and on esophageal motility. Manometry may record constant reductions in LES pressures (< 6 mm Hg) or altered peristalsis. Both events increase esophageal clearing time. It must however be remembered that in the development of GER transitory sphincter relaxation episodes also play an important role, and are more difficult to detect. Manometry, coupled with pH recordings, offers a precise functional outline of the esophagus, and may be useful in choosing candidates for surgery: altered esophageal motility contraindicates surgical correction [76]. The contribution of this test is quantitatively less important compared to other techniques [77]. Test positivity is recorded in 42%-52% of patients with demonstrated GER. The test may be negative in 30% of patients with esophagitis.

Esophageal pH monitoring is the principal technique in the diagnosis of GER. Reflux profile may be assessed by determining the number and time length of episodes over 24 hours, effect of body position (supine, combined), pH values (acid, alkaline, mixed), average esophageal pH over 24 hours and other parameters, as suggested by DeMeester et al. [78]. Prolonged computer-based pH monitoring shows the correlation between symptom onset (digestive or respiratory) and the reflux episodes. Portable instruments record esophageal, gastric, and duodenal endoluminal pH for 24 hours or more, in nearly physiological conditions, allowing the patient to conduct normal daily activities. This technique is considered the "gold standard" in the diagnosis of GER and allows recording the following information:

1. Presence of pathological reflux. It is well known that GER is not an "all or nothing" phenomenon but a physiological event also occurring in asymptomatic healthy subjects. An arbitrary cut-off has been chosen to discriminate between physiological and pathological reflux. Most authors now feel that the best discriminant is a fall in pH values below 4. However, our group has shown that, at least according to a good in vivo model of asthma such as sheep, the discriminant value could be lowered to pH < 3 [63]. The definition of the beginning and end of reflux activity, the minimal length of reflux time, and the best parameter for the global definition of GER might be still open to debate. It is now felt by some gastroenterologists that the best discriminant may be the time of acid exposure, calculated as the total time during which esophageal pH is below 4. This is in contrast with data showing that in GER-correlated asthma, differently from GER-correlated chronic bronchitis, this time could be very short [12].

2. If the GER episodes are the cause of a patient's symptoms. By means of pH monitoring a temporal association may be observed between diagnosed reflux episodes and respiratory symptoms.

3. If acid GER induces esophageal lesions. Although reports in the literature describe a good association between pH monitoring and esophagitis severity, this test cannot be considered conclusive in diagnosing derangements of the esophageal mucosa.

4. If treatment regimens reduce GER. Monitoring GER during treatment is possible and of great use in patients undergoing surgery (persistence of pathological reflux following fundoplication is apparently associated with a high risk of future clinical deterioration in patients who do not respond to treatment).

A further issue open to debate is the length of pH monitoring. Many authors have tested the diagnostic capabilities of recordings limited to a few hours, possibly in periods of the day during which reflux episodes are highly probable (after a meal, nocturnal). However, a critical review of the literature indicates that 24-hour recordings optimize sensitivity and specificity of the test. Reported sensitivity varies between 79% and 95% and specificity between 87% and 100%. It must also be underlined that the reproducibility of pH recordings is directly associated with the length of the test.

In recent literature new and interesting ideas have been suggested to add value to this diagnostic test. Jack et al. [79, 80] have performed concomitant recordings of esophageal and tracheal pH in asthmatic patients with GER, showing that at least some reflux episodes are followed by aspiration in the trachea with important acute modifications of respiratory function.

Evening gastroesophageal scintigraphy, followed with a pulmonary scintiscan the morning after (in most cases the patient ingests a liquid containing the Tc99m radionuclide) is a relatively recent test in the evaluation of patients with

GER for whom microaspiration of gastric substances into the airways is suspected. The test also gathers information on esophageal peristalsis and on gastric emptying time. It is a rapid, simple, noninvasive technique and can be repeated with little disturbance to the patient [81].

Esophageal scintigraphy may be particularly useful in diagnosing biliary reflux or gastric achlorhydria, situations not detectable by standard pH monitoring. There is no consensus on the true utility of this technique given its extremely high specificity but low sensitivity [76, 82]. For example, there is no correlation between scintiscan and pH monitoring results, even though both tests last many hours (up to 24 h). Tolia and Kuhns [83] compared concomitant pH monitoring and scintiscan recordings in 29 children with GER aged < 12 months. Scintiscans showed a higher sensitivity than pH monitoring in detecting reflux, particularly during the 60 minutes following a meal, whereas in other periods pH monitoring was more reliable. Suggestions have been made to increase test sensitivity, such as scintigraphic imaging every 10 seconds instead of every 30-60 seconds as is traditionally performed.

Of great importance are procedures that allow evaluation of the consequences of reflux activity:

Endoscopy. Modern, flexible fiber-optic instruments allow an accurate inspection of the esophageal surface, and biopsies may be performed for histologic evaluation. Endoscopy may be useful in determining the efficacy of antireflux therapy when employed in follow-up programs of patients undergoing conservative treatment or surgical procedures. Sontag et al. [46] found endoscopical evidence of esophagitis or Barrett's esophagus in 39% of 186 asthmatic patients.

The *Bernstein test* is technically simple and presents a high sensitivity [84]. It is performed by instilling diluted hydrochloric acid into the esophagus. The test is considered positive if the procedure evokes pain or heartburn within 10 minutes from the start of the test. Perpina et al.[85, 86] have shown that the instillation of 0.1 N hydrochloric acid may determine bronchoconstriction. The presence of low pH in the distal portion of the esophagus decreases the bronchial hyperreactivity threshold to histamine and methacholine. Schan et al. [53] showed that the presence of acid in the lower esophagus is associated with a fall in PEF in all patients tested as well as in controls. This response was not related to a positive or negative reaction for the Bernstein test and is therefore unrelated to inflammation of the esophageal mucosal lining. Moreover, asthmatic patiens with GER, contrarily to others, showed no improvement in PEF following correction of esophageal pH. The authors suggested that these patients may possess an exaggerated vagus-mediated reflex response, as expressed by altered parasympathetic reactivity of the airways.

Ultrasonography, a relatively recent technique for the diagnosis of GER, is nonirradiating, noninvasive and requires neither anesthesia nor sedation. According to some observations it demonstrates both anatomical changes such as hiatal hernia favoring GER and GER itself, especially in children whose symptoms can be effectively assessed in paraphysiologic conditions. The use of endoscopic ultrasonography has been also described in which the echographic probe is passed into the esophagus: this method appears optimal for staging the degree of severity of reflux esophagitis as well as its response to therapy [87]. For some authors, echographic techniques could be the future gold standard for assessing GER [88, 89], replacing pH monitoring as the principal analysis.

Treatment

Surprisingly, no more than fifteen studies on antireflux treatment in asthma patients with GER are present in peer-reviewed literature [90, 91]. Controlled studies have been conducted on alginates [92], H_2-receptor antagonists including cimetidine [16, 93] and ranitidine [94-96], cisapride [97] and, particularly, omeprazole [98, 103]. Concomitant and significant therapeutical efficacy on both esophageal and respiratory manifestations was observed in five studies (one each with cimetidine and ranitidine, and three with omeprazole).

In studies conducted by our group [99, 103] on omeprazole in asthma and GER, gas exchange parameters were analyzed in addition to traditional FEV1 and PEF values. Furthermore, bronchial response to methacholine was also assessed. Treatment was associated with clear-cut, significant functional improvement. To date, no controlled study has evaluated the effects of integrated treatment aimed at correcting specific defects (e.g. reflux of gastric material, its pH, and presence of esophageal dyskinesia) capable of causing reflux-induced asthma.

My colleagues and I are currently terminating an as yet unpublished study carried out on a vast population of subjects. Results appear promising both in terms of symptom control and functional improvement, not present in the previously quoted studies. In our study we observed asthmatic patients (n = 148) with hiatal hernia and GER. Treatment consisted of dietary restrictions, lifting the upper part of the bed, and administration of alginate-omeprazole. In patients with scintiscan demonstration of esophageal dyskinesia (21%), cisapride was also added. The results showed an improvement in respiratory symptoms, reduction in beta-2-agonist and steroid use, and a significant and relatively long-lasting functional improvement.

Dietary and daily habits that contribute to opposing GER must not be overlooked. The following should be avoided: gas-containing alcohol-based drinks (beer, champagne, sparkling wine), soft drinks, coffee, tea, chocolate, fatty meals, citrus fruits, bananas, tomatoes, garlic, mint, liquorice, and meat soup. Cigarette smoking must be interrupted, together with the habit of lying in bed or performing exercise after a meal. Weight control must be implemented, and tight belts or corsets should be avoided. The head and trunk should be raised when resting. Lastly, it must be remembered that most "respiratory" drugs exert a negative effect on the stomach (e.g. oral steroids, NSAID), or reduce LES competence (e.g. oral beta-2-agonists, theophylline) by relaxing esophageal smooth muscle fibers.

References

1. Winkelstein A (1935) Peptic esophagitis: a new clinical entity. JAMA 104:906-909
2. Allison PR (1946) Peptic ulcer of the esophagus. J Thorac Surg 15:308-317
3. Osler WB (1912) The principles and practice of medicine, 8th edn. D. Appleton, New York, pp 628-631
4. Clemencon GH, Osterman PO (1961) Hiatal hernia in bronchial asthma: the importance of concomitant pulmonary emphysema. Gastroenterology 95:110-120
5. Overholt RH, Ashraf MM (1966) Esophageal reflux as a trigger of asthma. NY State J Med 66:3030-3032
6. Danus O, Casar L, Latrain A, Pope CE II (1976) Esophageal reflux and unrecognized cause of recurrent obstructive bronchitis in children. J Pediatr 89:220-224
7. Christie DL, O'Grady LR, Mack DV (1978) Incompetent lower esophageal reflux in recurrent acute pulmonary disease of infancy and childhood. J Pediatr 93:23-27
8. Mansfield LE, Stein MR (1978) Gastroesophageal reflux and asthma: a possible reflex mechanism. Ann Allergy 41:224-226
9. Tuchman DN, Boyle JT, Pack AI, Schwartz J, Kokonos M, Spitzer AR, Cohen S (1984) Comparison of airway response following tracheal esophageal acidification in the cat. Gastroenterology 87:872-881
10. Hoyoux C, Forget T, Lambrich L, Geubelle F (1985) Chronic bronchopulmonary disease and gastroesophageal reflux in children. Pediatr Pulmonol 1:149-153
11. Gustafsson PM, Kjellman NI, Tibbling L (1986) Oesophageal function and symptoms in moderate and severe asthma. Acta Pediatr Scand 5:729-733
12. Ducoloné A, Vandevenne A, Jouin H, Grob JC, Coumaros D, Meyer C, Burghard G, Methlin G, Hollender L (1987) Gastroesophageal reflux in patients with asthma and chronic bronchitis. Am Rev Respir Dis 135:327-332
13. Crausaz FM, Favez G (1988) Aspiration of solid food particles into the lungs of patients with gastroesophageal reflux and chronic bronchial disease. Chest 93: 376-378
14. Perrin-Fayolle M (1990) Gastroesophageal reflux and chronic respiratory disease in adults: influence and results of surgical therapy. Clin Rev Allergy 8:457-469
15. Sontag SJ, O'Connel S, Khandelwal S, Miller T, Nemchausky B, Schnell TG, Serlovsky R (1990) Most asthmatics have gastroesophageal reflux with or without bronchodilator therapy. Gastroenterology 99:613-620
16. Larrain A, Carrasco E, Galleguillos F, Sepulveda R, Pope CE II (1991) Medical and surgical treatment of nonallergic asthma associated with gastroesophageal reflux. Chest 99:1330-1335
17. Donnelly RJ, Berrisford RG, Jack CI, Tran JA, Evans CC (1993) Simultaneous tracheal and esophageal pH monitoring: investigating reflux associated asthma. Ann Thorac Surg 56:1029-1033
18. Simpson WG (1995) Gastroesophageal reflux and asthma: diagnosis and management. Arch Intern Med 155:798-803
19. Harding SM, Richter JE, Guzzo MR, Schan G, Alexander RW, Bradley LA (1996) Asthma and gastroesophageal reflux: acid suppressive therapy improves asthma outcome. Am J Med 100:395-405
20. Moran TJ (1965) Experimental aspiration pneumonia: IV. Inflammatory and reparative changes produced by intratracheal injections of autologous gastric juice and hydrochloric acid. Arch Pathol 60:122-129
21. Pearson JEG, Wilson RSE (1971) Diffuse pulmonary fibrosis and hiatus hernia. Thorax 26:300-305

22. Sladen A, Zanca P, Hadnott WH (1971) Aspiration pneumonitis: the sequelae. Chest 59:448-450

23. Downs JB, Chapman RL, Modell JH, Hood CI (1974) An evaluation of steroid therapy in aspiration pneumonitis. Anesthesiology 40:129-135

24. Mays EE, Dubois JJ, Hamilton GB (1976) Pulmonary fibrosis associated with tracheobronchial aspiration: a study of the frequency of hiatal hernia and gastroesophageal reflux in interstitial pulmonary fibrosis of obscure etiology. Chest 69:512-515

25. Tobin RW, Pope CE II, Pellegrini CA, Emond MJ, Sillery J, Raghu G (1998) Increased prevalence of gastroesophageal reflux in patients with idiopathic pulmonary fibrosis. Am J Respir Care Med 158:1804-1808

26. Irwin RS, Corrao WM, Pratter MR (1981) Chronic persistent cough in the adult: the spectrum and frequency of causes and successful outcome of specific therapy. Am Rev Respir Dis 123:413-417

27. Irwin RS, Zawacki JK, Curley FJ, French CL, Hoffman P (1989) Chronic cough as the sole presenting manifestation of gastroesophageal reflux. Am Rev Respir Dis 140:1294-1300

28. Irwin RS, Curley FJ, French CL (1990) Chronic cough: the spectrum and frequency of causes, key components of the diagnostic evaluation, and outcome of the specific therapy. Am Rev Respir Dis 141:640-647

29. Ing AJ, Ngu MC, Breslin ABX (1994) The pathogenesis of chronic persistent cough associated with gastroesophageal reflux. Am J Respir Crit Care Med 149:160-167

30. Herbst JJ, Book LS, Bry PF (1978) Gastroesophageal reflux in the "near miss" sudden infant death syndrome. J Pediatr 92:73-75

31. Weiner GJ, Koufman JA, Wu WC, Cooper JB, Richter JE, Castell DO (1989) Chronic hoarseness secondary to gastroesophageal reflux disease: documentation with 24-h ambulatory pH monitoring. Am J Gastroenterol 84:1503-1508

32. Koufman JA (1991) The otolaryngologic manifestation of gastroesophageal disease. Laryngoscope 10[Suppl 53]:1-78

33. Cote DN, Miller RH (1995) The association of gastroesophageal reflux and otolaryngologic disorders. Compr Ther 21:80-84

34. Kambic V, Radsel Z (1984) Acid posterior laryngitis aetiology, histology diagnosis and treatment. J Laryngol Otol 98:1237-1240

35. Gaynor EB (1988) Gastroesophageal reflux as aetiologic factor in laryngeal complications of intubation. Laryngoscope 98:972-979

36. Jacob P, Kahrilas PJ, Herzon G (1991) Proximal esophageal pH-metry in patients with "reflux laryngitis". Gastroenterology 100:305-310

37. Kamel PL, Hanson D, Kahrilas PJ (1994) Prospective trial of omeoprazole in the treatment of posterior laryngitis. Am J Med 96:321-326

38. Hanson DG, Kamel PL, Kahrilas PJ (1995) Outcomes of anti-reflux therapy in the treatment of chronic laryngitis. Ann Otol Rhinol Laryngol 104:550-555

39. Cherry J, Margulies SI (1968) Contact ulcer of the larynx. Laryngoscope 78:1937-1940

40. Morrison MD (1988) Is chronic gastroesophageal reflux a causative factor in glottic carcinoma? Otolaryngol Head Neck Surg 99:370-373

41. Ward PH, Hanson DG (1988) Reflux as etiologic factor of carcinoma of the laryngopharynx. Laryngoscope 98:1195-1199

42. Savary M, Miller G (1977) Handbuch und Endoskopisches Atlas. Grassman Verlag, Solothurn (Schweitz)

43. Berquist VE, Rachelefski GS, Kadden M, Siegel SC, Katz RM, Fonkalsrud ES, Ament ME (1981) Gastroesophageal reflux associated with recurrent pneumonia and asthma in children. Pediatrics 68:29-35

44. Allen CJ, Craven MA, Waterfall WE, Newhouse MT (1989) Gastroesophageal reflux

and chronic respiratory disease. In: Baum G, Wolinsky E (eds) Textbook of pulmonary diseases, 4th edn. Little, Brown, Boston, pp 1471-1486

45. Chernow B, Castell DO (1977) Asthma and gastroesophageal reflux. JAMA 37:2379 (letter)
46. Sontag SJ, Schnell TG, Miller TQ, Khandelwal S, O'Connel S, Chejfee G, Greenlee H, Seidel UJ, Brand L (1992) Prevalence of oesophagitis in asthmatics. Gut 33:872-876
47. Bannister WK, Sattilaro AJ, Otis RD (1961) Therapeutic aspects of aspiration pneumonitis in experimental animals. Anesthesiology 22:440-443
48. Karlsson JA, Sant'Ambrogio G, Widdicombe J (1988) Afferent neural pathways in cough and reflex bronchoconstriction. J Appl Physiol 65:1007-1023
49. Cunningham ET Jr, Ravich WJ, Jones B, Donner MW (1992) Vagal reflexes referred from the upper aerodigestive tract: an infrequently recognized cause of cardiorespiratory response. Ann Intern Med 116:575-582
50. Ghaed N, Stein M (1979) Assessment of a technique for scintigraphic monitoring of pulmonary aspiration of gastric contents in asthmatics with gastroesophageal reflux. Ann Allergy 42:306-308
51. Greyson ND, Reid RH, Lin YC, Thomas P (1982) Radionuclide assessment in nocturnal asthma. Clin Nucl Med 7:318-319
52. Ruth M, Carlsson S, Mansson I, Bengtsson U, Sandberg N (1993) Scintigraphic detection of gastropulmonary aspiration in patients with respiratory disorders. Clin Physiol 13:19-33
53. Schan CA, Harding SM, Haile JM, Bradley LA, Richter JE (1994) Gastroesophageal reflux-induced bronchoconstriction: an intraesophageal acid infusion study using state-of-the art technology. Chest 106:731-737
54. Harding SM, Schan CA, Guzzo MR, Alexander RW, Bradley LA, Richter JE (1995) Gastroesophageal reflux-induced bronchoconstriction: is microaspiration a factor? Chest 108:1220-1227
55. Mansfield LE, Hameister HH, Spaulding HS, Smith NJ, Glab N (1981) The role of the vagus nerve in airway narrowing caused by intraesophageal hydrochloric acid provocative and esophageal distention. Ann Allergy 47:431-434
56. Spaulding HS Jr, Mansfield LE, Stein MR, Sellner JC, Gremillion DE (1982) Further investigation of the association between gastroesophageal reflux and bronchoconstriction. J Allergy Clin Immunol 69:516-521
57. Andersen LI, Schmidt A, Bundgaard A (1986) Pulmonary function and acid application in the esophagus. Chest 90:358-363
58. Harding SM, Guzzo MR, Maples R, Alexander RW, Richter E (1995) Gastroesophageal reflux induced bronchoconstriction: vagolytic doses of atropine diminish airway responses to esophageal acid infusion. Am J Respir Crit Care Med 151: A589 (abstract)
59. Hervé P, Denjean A, Jian R, Simonneau G, Duroux P (1986) Intraesophageal perfusion of acid increases the bronchomotor response to methacholine and to isocapnic hyperventilation in asthmatic subjects. Am Rev Respir Dis 134:986-989
60. Ekström T, Tibbling L (1989) Esophageal acid perfusion, airway function and symptoms in asthmatic patients with marked bronchial hyperreactivity. Chest 96:995-998
61. Allegra L, Tognella S (1997) Malattia da reflusso gastroesofageo ed asma. In: Allegra L (ed) Valutazione e gestione del paziente asmatico. Editeam, Castello d'Argile (Bologna), pp 23-27
62. Perrin-Fayolle M, Bel A, Kofman J, Harf R, Montagon B, Pacheco Y, Dandet J, Nessoz J, Perpoint B (1980) Asthma and gastroesophageal reflux. Results of the survey of over 150 cases. Poumon Coeur 36:225-230
63. Scuri M, Allegra L, Dal Negro RW, Pomari C, Abraham WM (1999) An ovine model

of GERD-induced bronchoconstriction. In: Dal Negro RW, Allegra L (eds) Pneumological aspects of gastroesophageal reflux. Springer, Milan, pp 43-52

64. Visconti A, Cuttitta G, Insalaco G, Peralta G, Catania G, Trizzino A, Bonsignore G (1990) Gastroesophageal reflux and nocturnal bronchoconstriction. In: Olivieri D, Bianco S (eds) Airway Obtruction and Inflammation. Progress Respir Res, vol. 24, Karger, Basel, pp 179-182

65. Depla AC (1989) Gastroesophageal reflux in patients with bronchial asthma. Digestion 44[Suppl 1]:63-67

66. Ekström T, Tibbling L (1989) Can mild bronchospasm reduce gastroesophageal reflux? Am Rev Respir Dis 139:52-55

67. Bartlett SG, Gorbach SL, Finegolo SM (1974) The bacteriology of aspiration pneumonia. Am J Med 56: 202-207

68. Lorber B, Swenson RM (1974) Bacteriology of aspiration pneumonia. A prospective study of community- and hospital-acquired cases. Ann Inter Med 81:329-331

69. Downing SE, Lee JC (1975) Laryngeal chemosensitivity: a possible mechanism for sudden infant death. Pediatrics 55:640-649

70. Harned HS, Myracle J, Ferriero J (1978) Respiratory suppression and swallowing from introduction of fluids into the laryngeal region of the lamb. Pediatr Res 12:1003-1009

71. Irwin RS, Curley FJ, French CL (1981) Chronic persistent cough in the adult: the spectrum and frequency of causes and successful outcome of specific therapy. Am Rev Respir Dis 123:413-417

72. Andze GO, Brandt ML, St Vil D, Bensoussan AL, Blanchard H (1991) Diagnosis and treatment of gastroesophageal reflux in 500 children with respiratory symptoms: the value of pH monitoring. J Pediatr Surg 26:295-300

73. Allegra L (1998) Asma e GERD. Aria Ambiente Salute 1(4):31-32

74. Allegra L (1999) Malattie respiratorie e reflusso gastroesofageo. Giorn It Mal Tor 53:15-22

75. Sondheimer JM (1998) Gasteroesophageal reflux: update on pathogenesis and diagnosis. Pediatr Clin North Am 35:103-116

76. Orenstein SR (1993) Gastroesophageal reflux. In: Wyllie R, Hyams JS (eds) Pediatric gastrointestinal disease: pathophysiology, diagnosis, management. WB Saunders, Philadelphia, pp 337-369

77. Welch RW, Luckmann K, Ricks P (1980) Lower esophageal sphincter pressure in histologic esophagitis. Dig Dis Sci 25:420-426

78. De Meester TR, Johnson LF, Joseph GJ, Toscano MS, Hall AW, Skinner DB (1976) Patterns of gastroesophageal reflux in health and disease. Ann Surg 184:459-470

79. Jack CIA, Walshaw MJ, Tran J, Hind CRK, Evans CC (1994) Twenty-four-hour tracheal pH monitoring - a simple and non-hazardous investigation. Respir Med 88:441-444

80. Jack CIA, Calverley PMA, Donnelly RJ, Tran J, Russel G, Hind CRK, Evans CC (1995) Simultaneous tracheal and esophageal pH measurements in asthmatic patients with gastro-esophageal reflux. Thorax 50:201-204

81. Gonzalez-Fernandez F, Arguelles-Martin F, Rodriguez de Quesada B (1987) Gastroesophageal scintigraphy: an useful screening test for GE reflux. J Pediatr Gastroenterol Nutr 6:217-219

82. Barish CF, Wu WC et al (1985) Respiratory complication of gastroesophageal reflux. Arch Intern Med 145:1882-1988

83. Tolia V, Kuhns L (1993) Comparison of simultaneous esophageal pH monitoring and scintigraphy in infants with gastroesophageal reflux. Am J Gastroenterol 88:661-664

84. Bernstein LM, Baker LA (1958) A clinical test for esophagitis. Gastroenterology 34:760-781

85. Perpina M, Ponce J, Marco V, Benlloch E, Miralbes M, Berenguer J (1983) The prevalence of asymptomatic gastroesophageal reflux in bronchial asthma and in non-asthmatic individuals. Eur J Respir Dis 64:582-587

86. Perpina M, Pellicer C, Marco V, Maldonado J, Ponce J (1985) The significance of the reflex bronchoconstriction provoked by gastroesophageal reflux in bronchial asthma. Eur J Respir Dis 66:91-97

87. Caletti GC, Ferrari A, Mattoli S, Zannoli R, Di Simone MB, Bocus P, Gozetti G, Barbara L (1997) Endoscopy vs ultrasonography in staging reflux esophagitis. Endoscopy 26:794-797

88. Westra SJ, Wolf BHM, Stealman CR (1990) Ultrasound diagnosis of gastroesophageal reflux and hiatus hernia in young children. J Clin Ultrasound 18:477-485

89. Westra SJ, Derkx HHF, Taminiau JA (1994) Symptomatic gastroesophageal reflux: diagnosis with ultrasound. J Pediatr Gastroenterol Nutr 19:58-64

90. Vigneri S, Termini R, Leandro G, Badalamenti S, Pantalena M, Savarino V, Di Mario F, Battaglia G, Mela GS, Pilotto A, Plebani M, Davì G (1995) A comparison of five maintenance therapies for reflux esophagitis. N Engl J Med 333:1106-1110

91. Field SK, Sutherland LR (1998) Does medical antireflux therapy improve asthma in asthmatics with gastroesophageal reflux? A critical review of the literature. Chest 114: 275-283

92. Kjellen G, Tibbling L, Wranne B (1981) Effect of conservative treatment of esophageal dysfunction on bronchial asthma. Eur J Respir Dis 62:190-197

93. Goodhall RJ, Earis JE, Cooper DN, Bernstein A (1981) Relationship between asthma and gastro-oesophageal reflux. Thorax 36:116-121

94. Harper PC, Bergren A, Kaye MD (1987) Anti-reflux treatment in asthma: improvement in patients with associated gastroesophageal reflux. Arch Intern Med, 147: 56-60

95. Ekström T, Lindgren BR, Tibbling L (1989) Effects of ranitidine treatment on patient with asthma and a history of gastro-oesophageal reflux: a double blind cross over study. Thorax 44:19-23

96. Gustafsson PM, Kjellman WIM, Tibbling L (1992) A trial of ranitidine in asthmatic children and adolescents with or without pathological gastroesophageal reflux. Eur Respir J 5:201-206

97. Tucci J, Resti M, Fontana R, Novembre E, Lami CA, Vierucci A (1993) Gastroesophageal reflux and bronchial asthma: prevalence and effect of cisapride therapy. J Pediatr Gastroenterol Nutr 17:265-270

98. Maton PN (1991) Omeprazole. N Engl J Med 324:965-975

99. Dal Negro RW, Pomari C, Turco P, Allegra L (1994) Gastroesophageal reflux and bronchial asthma: a cross-over omeprazole vs placebo comparison. Am J Respir Crit Care 149:A202 (abstract)

100. Meier JH, Mc Nally PR, Punja M, Freeman SR, Sudduth RH, Stocker N, Perry M, Spaulding HS (1994) Does omeprazole improve respiratory function in asthmatics with gastroesophageal reflux? A double-blind, placebo-controlled crossover study. Dig Dis Sci 39:2127-2133

101. Ford GA, Oliver PS, Prior JS, Butland RJ, Wilkinson SP (1994) Omeprazole in the treatment of asthmatics with nocturnal symptoms and gastro-oesophageal reflux: a placebo-controlled cross-over study. Postgrad Med J 70:350-354

102. Teichtal H, Kronborg IJ, Yeomans ND, Robinson P (1996) Adult asthma and gastro-oesophageal reflux: the effects of omeprazole therapy on asthma. Aust NZ J Med 26:671-676

103. Dal Negro R, Pomari C, Micheletto C, Turco P (1996) Omeprazole, but not placebo, reduces the bronchial response to methacholine in mild nonatopic asthmatics with gastroesophageal reflux. Am J Respir Crit Care Med 153:A517 (abstract)

Gastroesophageal Reflux in Chronic Obstructive Pulmonary Disease

M. LUSUARDI and C.F. DONNER

Introduction

The frequent association of gastroesophageal reflux (GER) and respiratory disorders, in particular asthma, chronic obstructive pulmonary disease (COPD), chronic dry cough, cystic fibrosis and idiopathic pulmonary fibrosis, is well known [1-4]. In this short review, the terms COPD and chronic bronchitis will be used indifferently to indicate a clinical picture characterized by chronic productive cough (for at least two months a year in the past two years) and possible bronchial obstruction with a significant irreversible component. The incidence of GER in asthma ranges from 40% to 80% according to the series; the figures for chronic bronchitis are about 50%-60% [1, 5]. In the study of Ducoloné et al. [5], about 50% of patients with GER had no clinical complaint of GER (although half of these had cough and nocturnal dyspnea) while the other 50% had both digestive and respiratory symptoms. Among the 17 subjects with GER, 9 were on theophylline treatment, but only 2 received sympathomimetic agents [5].

Causes and Risk Factors

The relationship between asthma or chronic dry cough and GER has been extensively investigated, but an exact cause-effect relationship is still a matter of debate [2]. In contrast, few studies in the literature have addressed the problem of the significance of GER in COPD. The issue is more complex than the GER-asthma relationship due to (a) the presence of a common risk factor such as smoking, and (b) the possibility of GER to be an isolated cause of chronic (dry) cough. Cigarette smoking can directly provoke acid reflux and exacerbate reflux disease, a possible mechanism being a long-lasting reduction of lower esophageal sphincter (LES) pressure causing an increased number of reflux events [6]. A

Division of Pulmonary Disease, Salvatore Maugeri Foundation, IRCCS, Rehabilitation Institute, Veruno (Novara), Italy

further possible mechanism is the prolongation of esophageal acid clearance time caused by a reduced buffering since smoking may alter salivary function [7]. The presence of both GER and COPD as concomitant but independent causes of chronic cough is often difficult to rule out, given the high prevalence of the two conditions.

As a further complication, drugs commonly used in COPD, such as xanthines and anticholinergic agents, may induce or aggravate GER. The mechanism behind this is related to a reduction of LES pressure [8]. Theophylline, but not enprophylline, is also prone to increase gastric secretions [9]. Despite this negative influence of drugs on GER, in a study of subjects with asthma and COPD it was not possible to differentiate patients with or without GER on the basis of bronchodilator treatment [5]. Studies on salbutamol administered either orally or by inhalation in normal subjects and asthma patients failed to demonstrate an effect on esophageal motility and GER during 24-hour pH monitoring [10, 11].

A negative influence on LES pressure in COPD may also be caused by mechanical reasons, i.e. a flattening of the diaphragm in a condition of pulmonary hyperinflation [12]. The importance of mechanical factors can be inferred from a study which, despite the limitation of comparing different conditions (COPD vs. asthma, chronic vs. acute conditions), demonstrated that the induction of bronchospasm in asthma increases the frequency and severity of GER episodes: one of the mechanisms proposed by the authors is that factors such as increased intrathoracic pressures, flattening of diaphragm and coughing reduce LES pressure and favor GER [13]. A more recent study on a group of asthmatic patients with GER submitted to histamine-challenge did not confirm that bronchospasm may worsen GER, notwithstanding theophylline treatment which per se clearly exacerbated GER [14].

Pathogenesis

While in many cases of asthma GER is recognized as an important trigger, if not a cause, and may have a pathogenetic role, in COPD GER does not seem equally important. Two different mechanisms of damage have been postulated in COPD, more by analogy with asthma and chronic nonproductive cough than by direct investigation: (1) microaspiration of esophageal contents into the tracheobronchial tree, and (2) an esophageal-tracheobronchial cholinergic reflex triggered by acidification of the distal esophagus [2].

Different studies have failed to show a bronchoconstrictive response to distal esophageal acidification in COPD patients, despite the fact that the patients experienced a significant increase in GER [5, 15]. Actually, Orr et al. showed that esophageal function in COPD is relatively normal [15], and concluded that reflex broncho-constriction seems to be unique to asthmatic patients [15]. These authors also studied the same patients during sleep and found that the acid infusion test did not cause an altered arousal response or latency to the first swallow, i.e. a normal arousal response with rapid swallowing allowed for prompt esophageal acid buffering [15].

An interesting hypothesis considers GER as a possible risk factor in COPD patients who have never smoked [1], through a mechanism of chronic microaspiration. Lung aspiration of acidic gastric contents is a known cause of pneumonia. GER with recurrent aspiration can be a cause of chronic pulmonary inflammation at least in recipients of heart-lung transplants [16]. Chronic microaspiration due to GER could well be a cause of chronic airways inflammation, which is the pathologic substrate of chronic bronchitis also in never-smokers [17], although a definitive demonstration has not been provided as yet. In a study on scintigraphic detection of gastropulmonary aspiration in 55 patients with chronic respiratory disorders and symptoms of GER, 11 patients were positive for aspiration, of whom only one had chronic bronchitis, 5 had asthma, 2 idiopathic chronic cough, 2 recurrent lung infection and 1 chronic laryngitis [18]. Interestingly, aspiration occurred indifferently in subjects with and without evidence of GER [18]. Two recent papers from the same group have stressed a possible role of swallowing disorders and consequent intermittent aspiration in causing chronic bronchitis in subjects with GER [19, 20]. Amelioration of respiratory symptoms was achieved after surgical intervention aimed at improving pharyngoesophageal function and swallowing; on the contrary no significant relief of cough and expectoration was obtained after treatment with a proton pump inhibitor [19, 20].

COPD on its own does not seem to influence the characteristics of GER, since no differences were found between subjects with chronic bronchitis and patients with digestive symptoms alone [5]. In a previous study, chronic bronchitics even showed a reduced frequency of GER episodes in comparison with patients with digestive symptoms alone [21]. On the other hand, GER induced by cough (stress reflux) was described some years ago in subjects with normal LES pressure and normal esophageal motility [22].

Treatment

A recent paper has readdressed the unresolved problem of reflux treatment with regard to respiratory symptoms in asthma and COPD [23]. COPD was defined in terms of irreversibility of baseline bronchial obstruction to a reversibility test with ipratropium bromide. Other characteristics of these COPD patients were similar to the asthmatic series, both groups having high bronchial hyperreactivity (BHR) despite chronic corticosteroid treatment by inhalation. The primary end point of the study was the effect of anti-reflux therapy on BHR. High dose omeprazole had a profound effect on reflux symptoms but no effect at all on BHR and secondary outcome measures [peak expiratory flow (PEF) variability, reversibility to ipratropium bromide, asthma symptoms and use of medications]. The authors concluded that, despite a high prevalence of GER in asthma and COPD, screening for GER and a general aggressive acid suppression therapy are not justified.

Conclusions

GER is frequently found in COPD, but only half of the patients with objective GER report digestive symptoms and GER treatment does not seem to modify respiratory symptoms. There is at present poor evidence of a cause-effect link between COPD and GER, even in those COPD patients with some clinical and functional characteristics similar to asthma (partially reversible airways obstruction, high BHR). A potential role of GER in COPD patients who have never smoked may be an interesting point for research. At present, the indication for a clinical investigation and treatment of GER in COPD patients, if any, seems largely independent of COPD itself.

References

1. Allen CJ, Newhouse MT (1984) Gastroesophageal reflux and chronic respiratory disease. Am Rev Respir Dis 129:645-647
2. Harding SM, Richter JE (1997) The role of gastroesophageal reflux in chronic cough and asthma. Chest 111:1389-1402
3. Ledson MJ, Wilson GE, Tran J, Walshaw MJ (1998) Tracheal microaspiration in adult cystic fibrosis. J R Soc Med 91:10-12
4. Mays EE, Dubois JJ, Hamilton GB (1976) Pulmonary fibrosis associated with tracheobronchial aspiration. Chest 69:512-515
5. Ducoloné A, Vandevenne A, Jouin H, Grob J-C, Coumaros D, Meyer C, Burghard G, Methlin G, Hollender L (1987) Gastroesophageal reflux in patients with asthma and chronic bronchitis. Am Rev Respir Dis 135:327-332
6. Kahrilas PJ, Gupta RR (1990) Mechanisms of acid reflux associated with cigarette smoking. Gut 31:4-10
7. Kahrilas PJ (1992) Cigarette smoking and gastroesophageal reflux disease. Dig Dis 10:61-71
8. Berquist WE, Rachelefsky GS, Kadden M, Siegel SC, Katz RM, Mickey MR, Ament ME (1981) Effect of theophylline on gastroesophageal reflux in normal adults. J Allergy Clin Immunol 67:407-411
9. Johannesson N, Andersson K-E, Joelsson B, Persson CGA (1985) Relaxation of lower esophageal sphincter and stimulation of gastric secretion and diuresis by antiasthmatic xanthines. Role of adenosine antagonism. Am Rev Respir Dis 131:26-31
10. Schindlbeck NE, Heinrich C, Huber RM, Muller-Lissner SA (1998) Effects of albuterol (salbutamol) on esophageal motility and gastroesophageal reflux in healthy volunteers. JAMA 260:3156-3158
11. Michoud MC, Leduc T, Proulx F, Perreault S, Du Souich P, Duranceau A, Amyot R (1991) Effect of salbutamol on gastroesophageal reflux in healthy volunteers and patients with asthma. J Allergy Clin Immunol 87:762-767
12. Roussos C, Macklem PT (1982) The respiratory muscles. N Engl J Med 307:786-797
13. Moote DW, Lloyd DA, McCourtie DR, Wells GA (1986) Increase in gastroesophageal reflux during methacholine-induced bronchospasm. J Allergy Clin Immunol 78:619-623
14. Ekstrom TKA, Tibbling LIE (1989) Can mild bronchospasm reduce gastroesophageal reflux? Am Rev Respir Dis 139:52-55

15. Orr WC, Shamma-Othman Z, Allen M, Robinson MG (1992) Esophageal function and gastroesophageal reflux during sleep and waking in patients with chronic obstructive pulmonary disease. Chest 101:1521-1525

16. Reid KR, McKenzie FN, Menkis AH, Novick RJ, Pflugfelder PW, Kostuk WJ, Ahmad D (1990) Importance of chronic aspiration in recipients of heart-lung transplants. Lancet 336:206-208

17. Lusuardi M, Capelli A, Cerutti CG, Spada EL, Donner CF (1994) Airways inflammation in subjects with chronic bronchitis who have never smoked. Thorax 49:1211-1216

18. Ruth M, Carlsson S, Mansson I, Bengtsson U, Sandberg N (1993) Scintigraphic detection of gastro-pulmonary aspiration in patients with respiratory disorders. Clin Physiol 13:19-33

19. Tibbling L (1993) Wrong-way swallowing as a possible cause of bronchitis in patients with gastroesophageal reflux disease. Acta Otolaryngol (Stockh) 113:405-408

20. Tibbling L, Gibellino FM, Johansson KE (1995) Is mis-swallowing or smoking a cause of respiratory symptoms in patients with gastroesophageal reflux disease? Dysphagia 10:113-116

21. David P, Denis P, Nouvet G, Pasquis G, Lefrancois R, Morere P (1982) Fonction respiratoire et reflux gastro-oesophagien au cours de la bronchite chronique. Bull Eur Physiopathol Respir 18:81-86

22. Pellegrini CA, DeMeester TR, Johnson LF, Skinner DB (1979) Gastroesophageal reflux and pulmonary aspiration: incidence, functional abnormality, and results of surgical therapy. Surgery 86:110-119

23. Boeree MJ, Peters FTM, Postma DS, Kleibeuker JH (1998) No effect of high-dose omeprazole in patients with severe airway hyperresponsiveness and (a)symptomatic gastro-oesophageal reflux. Eur Respir J 11:1070-1074

Gastroesophageal Reflux and Interstitial Lung Disease

E. Marangio and D. Olivieri

Introduction

Gastroesophageal reflux (GER) is an abnormal condition which causes the gastrointestinal contents to return to the esophagus, owing to alterations in the mechanisms which control gastroesophageal continence function [1].

Bronchial asthma is exacerbated by multiple triggers that produce contraction of the bronchial smooth muscles, mucous hypersecretion, and inflammatory responses with cell recruitment and mediator release. One of the most common, though often undervalued stimuli, is GER which, according to several studies, is prevalent in 40%-50% of asthma patients [2, 3].

Symptoms of disease caused by reflux are either esophageal or extra-esophageal manifestations, and include gastric, oropharyngeal, respiratory and thoracic symptoms. Respiratory manifestations associated with GER include a large group of symptoms and diseases such as sinusitis, pharyngitis, aphonia, laryngitis, laryngeal stenosis, whooping cough, dyspnea, chronic obstructive pulmonary diseases, bronchial asthma, bronchiectasis, ab ingestis pneumonia, relapsing pneumonia and lung fibrosis [4, 5].

Gastroesophageal Reflux Mechanisms

The smooth muscles of the lower third of the esophagus are organized into two longitudinal and circular layers, forming the lower esophagus sphincter (LES). The LES, together with the His angle and the esophagus diaphragmatic orifice, acts as a barrier which under normal conditions impedes reflux. Moreover, GER is a normal phenomenon which, although infrequent, acidic and short lived, usually occurs during and following meals. The severity of GER is directly related to gastric pH, quantity of material and the amount of contact refluxed material has with the esophageal mucus. Also, GER severity is inversely related to esophageal clearing capacity.

Institute of Respiratory Disease, University of Parma, Italy

The mechanism by which GER induces bronchial pulmonary diseases is not completely understood. However, two different hypotheses have recently been proposed:

(a) A *reflux* mechanism which directly aspirates the refluxed gastric contents into the lower airways [6];

(b) A *reflex* mechanism, by which the reflux of the gastric contents limited to the lower third of the esophagus causes bronchial spasms and modification of airway resistance by the activation of the vagal reflex [7].

During the reflux mechanism, the aspiration of gastric contents occurs by silent microaspiration. Interestingly, studies on animals show that the introduction of an acid solution (hydrochloric acid) for several minutes into the trachea or bronchi causes broncho-constriction and increased pulmonary resistance even in non-asthmatics [8]. This effect is short lived, vagally mediated and completely inhibited by vagotomy.

Another mechanism by which GER induces respiratory manifestations might be aspiration of gastric contents into the pharynx, causing stimulation of irritant receptors. In this regard, animal experiments showed that stimulation of the upper airway receptors with acid solution induces broncospasm [9]. However, in GER patients, receptor irritation is secondary to the stimulation of distal esophageal receptors. In this regard studies with radioisotopes were conducted in order to demonstrate microaspiration of the gastric contents into the lung in humans. The radioisotopes were instilled directly into the stomach through a nasogastric tube, and thorax radioactivity was successfully evaluated after a set time period.

These studies, however, demonstrated high specificity and low sensitivity, and they probably underestimated the importance of microaspiration [10]. An indirect method, with a pH electrode located directly under the upper esophageal sphincter, demonstrated that patients with reflux at this level have an elevated risk of aspiration, especially at night when sphincter pressure is reduced [11]. Other results from the literature indicate that the aspiration of gastric material containing hydrochloric acid and food, such as animal and vegetable fats, causes lung parenchyma inflammation, which can manifest as acute bacterial pneumonia. Additionally, over time aspiration can cause pulmonary abscesses, bronchiectasis and diffuse or local interstitial lung fibrosis [12]. Moreover, prolonged acid exposure in the proximal esophagus may be one of the pathogenetic factors of idiopathic pulmonary fibrosis (IPF) [13].

During the reflex mechanism, refluxed gastric material stimulates esophageal receptors by activation of a vagal reflex, which produces bronchospasm and modification of airway resistance. The finding that vagotomy completely abolishes bronchospasm induced by the infusion of acid into the esophagus in animals confirms the importance of the esophageal chemo-receptors. Additionally, studies in humans showed that acid infusion causes slight reduction of the forced expiratory volume in 1 s (FEV_1), while pre-medication with atropin prevents this effect, thus suggesting a possible role for vagal reflex [14].

Respiratory Manifestations

Although many studies have documented the correlation between GER, bronchial asthma and otorhinolaryngeal diseases, few studies have been made - mostly in pediatrics - on the relationship between GER and other respiratory manifestations. Since GER frequently occurs in children with respiratory disease, reflux may play a role in sudden infant death syndrome (SIDS), laryngospasm, bronchial asthma, aspiration pneumonia and recurrent pneumonia [15]. Owing to its particular etiopathogenic characteristics, aspiration pneumonia represents a peculiar type of pneumonia in children that presupposes the existence of predisposing factors such as GER, alterations in the state of consciousness, extraneous objects and immune alterations. Aspiration of gastric material into the lung parenchyma can cause various manifestations which differ according to the quantity and type of material and whether or not the aspiration is massive or chronic.

In adults, aspiration pneumonia is the most common illness caused by GER. This manifestation generally affects alcoholics, the immune-depressed, and weak hospitalized subjects with chronic illnesses (cardiorespiratory, renal, metabolic) or alterations in the state of consciousness [16, 17]. This condition is frequently caused by anaerobic, gram-negative bacteria and is generally the consequence of oropharyngeal flora aspiration. During aspiration pneumonia, acute necrosis occurs mainly in the center lobe; the bronchioles are often destroyed and substituted by acute inflammation with necrosis. Multinucleated giant cells are also present that phagocytize foreign materials. Moreover, sometimes granulomas from foreign bodies are also present.

Massive aspiration of gastric acid (pH lower than 3) produces diffuse alveolar damage (DAD) associated with intra-alveolar hemorrhage, pulmonary edema and necrosis of alveolar cells, namely Mendelson's syndrome [18, 19]. Although DAD is usually an acute manifestation, it nevertheless denotes the tendency of lung parenchyma to react, by causing fibrosis, to a pathogenic event which previously had not been correctly treated. Two distinct phases occur during DAD development:

(a) An early and exudative stage which occurs primarily during the first week, with edema and hyaline membranes;

(b) A later proliferative or organizing stage which occurs after 1-2 weeks whereby the tissue organizes and evolves towards fibrosis [18].

The earliest signs of the acute phase are evident after 12-24 h, and include intra-alveolar and interstitial edema with variable levels of intra-alveolar hemorrhage and fibrin deposition. Hyaline membranes develop during successive days and reach maximum levels 3-7 days from DAD inception. The membranes appear as homogeneous eosinophilic structures which deposit along the alveolar septa. They are usually accompanied by proteinaceous exudate containing cellular debris. Cell necrosis, which mostly affects the most vulnerable type-1 pneumocytes, causes the separation of the cells from the alveolar basal membrane, associated with areas of alveolar collapse. Frequently, in the interstitium, a variable level of inflammation can be seen where the lymphocytes, plasma cells and macrophages predominate. At the end of the acute phase, type-2 pneumocytes, which are more resistant to damage, show cell hyperplasia. This phenomenon is a reparatory reaction which continues into the succeeding phase. Additionally, these cells can differentiate into type-1 pneumocytes. Furthermore the bronchial epithelium is also commonly injured in DAD. In the early stage, epithelium cell necrosis occurs and at a later time, regeneration takes place with possible squamous metaplasia.

The organizing stage of DAD begins after one or more weeks, but is most important two weeks following injury. It is characterized by the proliferation of fibroblasts, and occurs principally in the interstitium. Moreover, interstitial inflammation and cell hyperplasia continue. The hyaline membranes are usually phagocytosed by the alveolar macrophages, while residual alveolar exudate can be incorporated inside the thickening alveolar septa. Fibrosis is localized around the alveolar ducts and, in the worst cases, can continue for several weeks and modify the parenchyma to form "honeycomb" lung.

To date, even though neutrophils are thought to have a central role, the mechanism which leads to DAD has not been fully understood. These cells, which are recruited by various chemotactic agents and stimulated by the activated complement system, probably accumulate in the lung capillaries, where they damage the endothelium by releasing enzymes such as elastases as well as oxidant radicals, thus involving inflammatory cells and amplifying responses. In this initial phase, an important role is played by the various cytokines such as tumor necrosis factor (TNF) and interleukin (IL) in regulating the formation and maintenance of damage. These cells that release other activating factors such as platelet-derived growth factor (PDGF), basic fibroblast growth factor (BFGF) and fibronectin probably cause successive fibroblast proliferation.

If damage is not diffuse but is localized at the peribronchiolar parenchyma, the diagnosis is bronchiolitis obliterans organizing pneumonia (BOOP). Interestingly, recurrent aspiration of gastric acid related to esophageal dysfunction and hiatal hernia, have been shown to induce BOOP and may be associated with interstitial lung fibrosis [20]. Patch fibrosis involving the bronchiolar lumen and the peribronchiolar airspaces is the histologic feature which characterizes BOOP. The presence of fibroblasts embedded in a myxoid matrix, rich in mucopolysaccharide acids, characterizes this type of fibrosis. Besides fibroblasts, various degrees of inflammation are present with lymphocytes, macrophages, plasma cells and neutrophils. Matrix and cells form plugs that occlude distal bronchioles, alveolar ducts and adjacent alveolar spaces. The accumulation of foamy lipid-containing macrophages, present in a type of alveolitis caused by bronchiolar occlusion, is also frequently seen. Lastly, owing to inflammation, the alveolar septa are usually thickened.

Controversy remains about whether chronic aspiration of gastric acid, which can occur in patients with gastroesophageal reflux, hiatal hernia or esophageal diverticula, causes interstitial lung diseases. Evidence exists which links GER with bronchial asthma and other airway pathologies such as chronic bronchitis and bronchiectasis [2, 3, 21]. Although several authors observed an association between idiopathic pulmonary fibrosis and GER, a direct causal relationship has not been demonstrated [22-24]. Recently, in this regard, it has been observed that patients with IPF, without typical GER symptoms, have increased acid exposure time in the proximal esophagus. Increased exposure may be related to the nocturnal supine position. This mechanism could suggest a significant role of GER in the pathogenesis of the IPF [13].

In order to highlight lung damage caused by chronic aspiration of gastric material related to GER, and to identify a possible specific lesion index, brochoalveolar lavage, bronchial aspirate, the cytologic examination of sputum and esophageal pH monitoring are used [12, 13, 25, 26]. Moreover, although clinical studies have been principally carried out in children, the presence of foamy lipid-containing macrophages has also been observed in adults [27, 28]. Even though a high number of cells could correlate with aspiration, this finding should not be considered specific. In this regard, while the absence of foamy lipid-containing macrophages is evidence against aspiration, their presence, although abundant, is also indicative of other diseases.

We should also keep in mind that macrophages can accumulate in the alveoli, and once activated can trigger inflammatory responses. Moreover, the persistence of this condition and the release of cytokines might explain the involvement and activation of fibroblasts in the interstitium, as well as the consequent evolution of the inflammatory process into fibrosis.

Conclusion

The real importance of GER as a cause of interstitial lung disease is difficult to evaluate. In addition, studies that have hypothesized the link between the two are dated and based on methods which have proved inadequate for the evaluation of GER. Lastly, since many patients do not manifest any disturbances, the subjective manifestation of reflux seems to be an inaccurate index of GER.

References

1. Roncoroni L (1994) Reflusso gastroesofageo ed esofagite. In: Okolicsanyi L, Peracchia A (eds) Malattie dell'apparato gastrointestinale, vol. 6. McGraw-Hill, Milano, pp 49-53
2. Sontag SJ, Schnell TG, Miller TQ, Khandelwal S, O'Connell S, Chejfec G, Greenlee H, Seidel UJ, Brand L (1992) Prevalence of esophagitis in asthmatics. Gut 33:872-876
3. Duclone A, Vandevenne A, Jouin H, Grob JC, Coumaros D, Meyer C, Burghard G, Methlin G, Hollender L (1987) Gastroesophageal reflux in patients with asthma and chronic bronchitis. Am Rev Respir Dis 135:327-332
4. el-Serag HB, Sonnenberg A (1997) Comorbid occurrence of laryngeal or pulmonary disease with esophagitis in United States military veterans. Gastroenterology 113:755-760
5. Ceccatelli P, Angioli D (1995) Malattia da reflusso gastroesofageo e patologia respi-

ratoria. In: Morelli A, Fiorucci S (eds) Malattia da reflusso gastroesofageo. EdiSES, Napoli, pp 210-221

6. Goldman JM, Bennett JR (1990) Gastroesophageal reflux and asthma: a common association, but of what clinical importance? Gut 31:1-3

7. Mansfield LE, Stein MR (1978) Gastroesophageal reflux and asthma: a possible reflex mechanism. Ann Allergy 41:224-226

8. Lyndon E, Mansfield (1989) Gastroesophageal reflux and disease of the respiratory tract: a review. J Asthma 26:271-278

9. Wynne JW, Ramphal R, Hood CI (1981) Tracheal mucosal damage after aspiration: a scanning electron microscope study. Am Rev Respir Dis 124:728-732

10. Ghaed N, Stein MR (1979) Assessment of a technique for scintigraphic monitoring of pulmonary aspiration of gastric contents in asthmatics with gastro-oesophageal reflux. Ann Allergy 42:306-308

11. Kahrilas PJ, Dodds WJ, Dent J, Haeberle B, Hogan WJ, Arndorfer RC (1987) Effects of sleep, spontaneous gastroesophageal reflux, and a meal on upper esophageal sphincter pressure in normal human volunteers. Gastroenterology 92:466-478

12. Corwin RW, Irwin RS (1985) The lipid-laden alveolar macrophage as a marker of aspiration in parenchymal lung disease. Am Rev Respir Dis 132:575-581

13. Tobin RW, Pope CE, Pellegrini CA, Edmond MJ, Sillery J, Raghu G (1998) Increased prevalence of gastroesophageal reflux in patients with idiopathic pulmonary fibrosis. Am J Respir Crit Care Med 158:1804-1808

14. Wright RA, Millar SA, Corsello BF (1990) Acid-induced esophago-bronchial-cardiac reflexes in humans. Gastroenterology 99:71-73

15. Fregonese B, Battistini E, Sacco O, Barabino A, Mattioli G (1998) Reflusso gastroesofageo e apparato respiratorio. In: Rossi G (ed) Pneumologia pediatrica (Collana di patologia pediatrica). McGraw-Hill, Milano, pp 421-424

16. Potgieter PD, Hammond JMJ (1992) Etiology and diagnosis of pneumonia requiring ICU admission: a discussion. Chest 101:199-203

17. Torres A, Serra-Batles J, Ferrer A, Jimenez P, Celis R, Cobo E, Rodriguez-Roisin R (1991) Severe community-acquired pneumonia: epidemiology and prognostic factors. Am Rev Respir Dis 144:312-318

18. Katzenstein A, Askin L (1997) Katzenstein and Askin's surgical pathology of non-neoplastic lung disease, 3rd edn. WB Saunders, Philadelphia, pp 417-437

19. James CE, Modell JH (1983) Pulmonary aspiration. Semin Anesth 2:177

20. Gosink BB, Friedman PJ, Liebow AA (1973) Bronchiolitis obliterans, Roentgenologic-pathologic correlation. Am J Roentgenol Radium Ther Nucl Med 117:816-832

21. David P, Denis P, Nouvet G, Pasquis P, Lefrancois R, Morere P (1982) Lung function and gastroesophageal reflux during chronic bronchitis. Bull Eur Physiopathol Respir 18:81-86

22. Allen CJ, Newhouse MT (1984) Gastroesophageal reflux and chronic respiratory disease. Am Rev Respir Dis 129:645-647

23. Pearson JEG, Wilson RES (1971) Diffuse pulmonary fibrosis and hiatus hernia. Thorax 26:300-305

24. Mays EE, Dubois JJ, Hamilton GB (1976) Pulmonary fibrosis associated with tracheobronchial aspiration. Chest 69:512-515

25. Wolfe JE, Bone RC, Ruth WE (1976) Diagnosis of gastric aspiration by fiberoptic bronchoscopy. Chest 70:458-459

26. Donnelly RJ, Berrisford RG, Jack CI, Tran A, Evans CC (1993) Simultaneous tracheal and esophageal pH monitoring: investigating reflux-associated asthma. Ann Thorac Surg 56:1029-1033

27. Collins KA, Geisinger KR, Wagner PH, Blackburn KS, Washburn LK, Block SB
     (1995) The cytologic evaluation of lipid-laden alveolar macrophages as an indicator
     of aspiration pneumonia in young children. Arch Pathol Lab Med 119:229-231
28. Langston C, Pappin A (1996) Lipid-laden alveolar macrophages as an indicator of
     aspiration pneumonia. Arch Pathol Lab Med 120:326

Diagnostic Techniques
for Gastroesophageal Reflux Detection

Imaging of Gastroesophageal Reflux

A. Michelon[1], M. Penini[1], and P.G. Giorgetti[2]

Introduction

Despite new imaging and endoscopic techniques, the study of the esophagus using barium contrast medium continues to be the fundamental radiographic analysis used for research into gastroesophageal reflux. Before illustrating how these techniques work, it is worth recalling some basic notions of esophageal anatomy.

The top of the esophagus is situated in the area of the sixth cervical vertebra at the point of the upper esophageal sphincter alongside Killian's mouth. The esophageal tract thus reaches the mediastinum (esophageal body or tubular segment). This tract, characterised by exclusively peristaltic activity, terminates just a few centimetres above the hiatus of the diaphragm. The esophagus passes through this into the abdomen, forming the vestibular area which then becomes the cardias at the tenth thoracic vertebra. While at rest, this last section is in a state of constant tonic contraction. It is a high manometric pressure area, controlled by the vagus nerve.

The vestibule can in turn be divided into three segments:

(i)   A section above the diaphragm, known as the epiphrenic ampulla, extending upwards as far as Schatzki's ring A (marking the transition from the tubular esophagus to the vestibular esophagus) and downwards as far as the lower esophageal sphincter.

(ii) An intermediate intra-hiatal segment.

(iii) A section below the diaphragm connecting with the stomach at the cardial orifice. This is the point of transition from the esophageal mucus to the gastric mucus, a point known by endoscopists as the "Z line". X-rays can sometimes trace this line when, in the presence of a trans-hiatal hernia, it is found above the diaphragm, showing up in the form of a small incisure also called Schatzki's ring B. Situated at precisely this junction of esophagus and stomach is an acute angle of His, one of the main anti-reflux

[1]Radiological Department, Bussolengo General Hospital, Bussolengo (Verona), Italy; [2]Nuclear Medicine Department, City General Hospital, Verona, Italy

mechanisms. The partial or total absence of this angle - together with hypotony of the lower esophageal sphincter - is the chief cause of gastroesophageal reflux. The precise physiological mechanism controlling the state of activity of the sphincter has not yet been clearly identified and is currently a controversial issue.

Research Methods

The now standard radiographic technique for a contrastographic study of the esophagus - dual contrast esophagography - is applied in two stages and involves intravenous injection of muscle relaxants (*N*-hyoscine butylbromide). In the first stage the patient, in an upright position, is given approximately 100 ml highly-concentrated, low-viscous barium suspension, at carefully monitored time intervals. The purpose of this is to create a satisfactory, uniform spread of the esophageal mucus. The "dual contrast" effect can be achieved in one of two ways: either by asking the patient to swallow air keeping the nostrils closed, or by administering effervescent powder together with a little water.

A number of scopically controlled radiograms are then carried out (either using rapid serial imaging or video recording, at different angles: antero-posterior, latero-lateral, oblique). These provide information regarding (i) the patency and plasticity of the esophageal lumen, (ii) its peristaltic activity, and (iii) the presence or absence of variations in the mucus and in the esophageal walls, such as ulcerative or vegetative lesions, diverticular formations, and *ab estrinseco* compressions.

In the second stage of the experiment the patient is asked to lie face down with the weight shifted to the right side (to avoid obstruction by the vertebral column), and then to assume the Trendelenburg position (X-ray position inclined by 10°-15°). In this position the progression of the barium meal is not affected by gravitational factors, thus allowing a more revealing evaluation of efficiency of the esophageal peristalsis, and highlighting even slight functional pathologies not detectable in the upright position. The face-down position enables the barium meal to collect in the lower gastric area and at the gastroesophageal junction, where, if there is malfunctioning of the closing mechanisms of the lower esophageal sphincter, a reflux may occur. This reaction is easily traced on the monitor and may also be recorded radiographically by means of a rapid series of seriograms, or by using a spot-camera with a frequency of 1-2 photograms per second (Fig. 1a,b).

Compressing the patient's abdomen (by applying pressure with a pillow) may help to make the reflux more evident, as will swallowing and taking a deep breath while making strenuous movements. As well as the reflux, other reactions may be provoked: (i) widening of the esophageal hiatus of the diaphragm, (ii) dislocation above the diaphragm of the esophageal-gastric junction, and (iii) the presence of trans-hiatal hernias and possibly their reducibility.

Over time the reflux of gastric juice into the esophagus can produce secon-

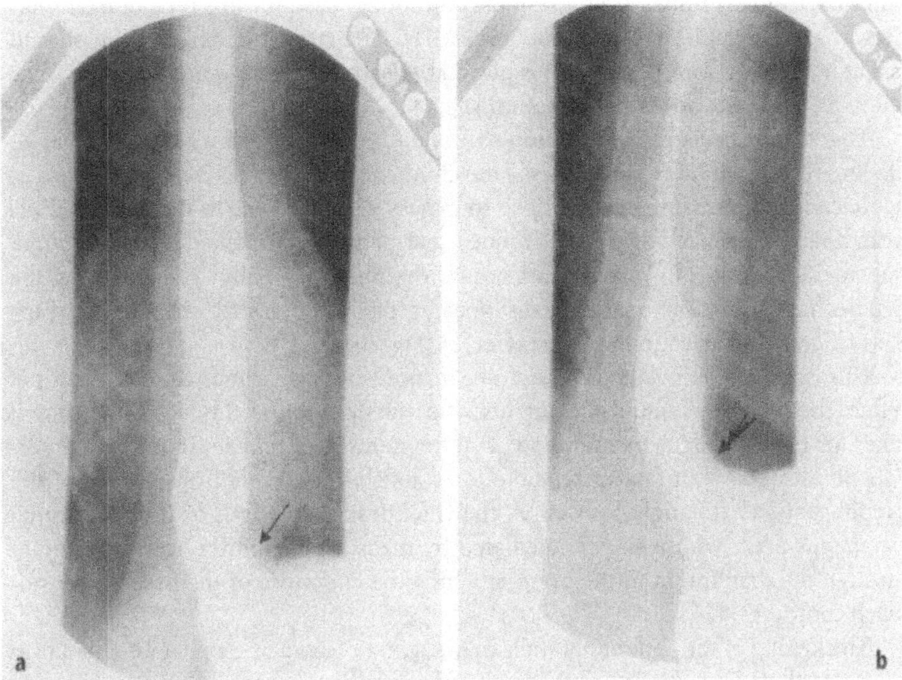

Fig. 1a,b. The reduction of the angle of His (*arrows*) causes the loss of one of the two main anti-reflux mechanisms - this involves the rising of the barium meal along the esophagus (with patient in clinostatic position)

dary esophagitis, detectable esophagraphically only in its most advanced stages, when changes in the make-up of the mucus may be recognised. These changes consist in thin linear images of refilling defects, and are associated with the presence of small incisures resulting from cicatricial retraction. In these cases, partly in view of possible phlogistic pathology, the diagnostic procedure must be completed by means of esophagoscopy and esophageal biopsy.

For infants and young children a further imaging technique - ultrasonography - may be adopted as an alternative to the traditional contrastographic study using barium meal. It should be underlined that children are particularly prone to this type of affection which, as well as causing respiratory difficulties, can retard growth. The problem stems from the fact that in children the angle of His is considerably less acute than in adults, and in some cases is not present at all. Consequently there is a practically uninterrupted connection between the esophagus and the stomach, which is therefore more subject to the onset of reflux. This takes the form of substantial regurgitations or vomiting immediately after meals.

The ultrasound analysis should be performed on a full stomach. Infants are fed a good quantity of milk, older children fruit juice. With the patient lying in a supine position, longitudinal scanning is effected on the esophageal-gastric junction. Convex probes are those most commonly used for this type of examination, with a variable frequency of 3.5-5 MHz. The real-time observation should last at least 10-15 min. The probe is placed beneath the xiphoid area, slightly rotated in an a counterclockwise direction [1].

The esophageal-gastric junction shows up in the shape of a tube, with variable length (depending on the age of the child examined) of 1.5-3 cm. It consists of hypoechogenous-shaped walls whose thickness varies from 1 to 2 mm. The walls form the boundary of a hyperechogenous central area (constituted by the lumen of the stomach) (Fig. 2a). When reflex occurs the muscular walls widen, causing the hyperechogenous central area to disappear, replaced by gastric substances which pass from the stomach to the esophagus [2] (Fig. 2b).

Ultrasound is of invaluable assistance in assessing the various characteristics of reflux: the volume of liquid flowing back up, the duration of the reflux, the time it takes for the esophagus to empty out, and the number of refluxes in the time intervals monitored [1]. It is also possible to establish the presence or absence of the esophageal-gastric angle, as well as the thickness and length of the abdominal esophagus area (whose size is calculated by measuring from the transition point through the diaphragm to the point at which the curvature of the base of the stomach continues) [2].

Thickening of the abdominal walls may suggest secondary esophagitis (the ultrasound method, however, is not the most efficient way of evaluating this; endoscopic analysis and biopsy – as with adults – should be used as a follow-up). Measuring is effected on the back wall, the one statistically most affected by phlogistic phenomena. Thickness exceeding 2-3 mm strongly suggests esophagitis [2]. Ultrasonography can also detect the presence of any associated trans-hiatal hernia [3].

Ultrasound may be adopted in unison with the barium meal radiographic method, but has the advantage of being able to capture information not otherwise obtainable (such as the thickness of the esophageal walls) [1]. It is also harmless (ionising radiation as a source of energy is not utilised), thus allowing much longer periods of observation [2, 3]. Moreover the meal offered to children is undoubtedly consumed more readily than the barium meal, thus facilitating the smooth running of the experiment. In consideration of these advantages, the ultrasound method may provide a good initial examination in screening gastroesophageal reflux, as well as an option for therapeutic follow-up in infants and young children.

Contrastographic radiography becomes necessary when accurate echography is impeded by a build-up of gas in the stomach, or when a more complete analysis of the whole esophagus is required, as is the case when inflammation occurs (such as esophagitis or esophageal stenosis).

Finally, gastroesophageal reflux can also be explored by means of scintigraphic examination as an imaging technique. Scintigraphic evaluation of esophageal-gastric transit and gastroesophageal reflux represents a good option inasmuch as it is noninvasive and totally physiological, requires low quantities of irradiation, is reasonably inexpensive, and may be used in a number of different clinical and therapeutic contexts owing to the possibility of quantifying the data obtained. It also enables those conducting the experiment to make a separate evaluation of the esophageal-gastric activity of solids and liquids using different types of food [4].

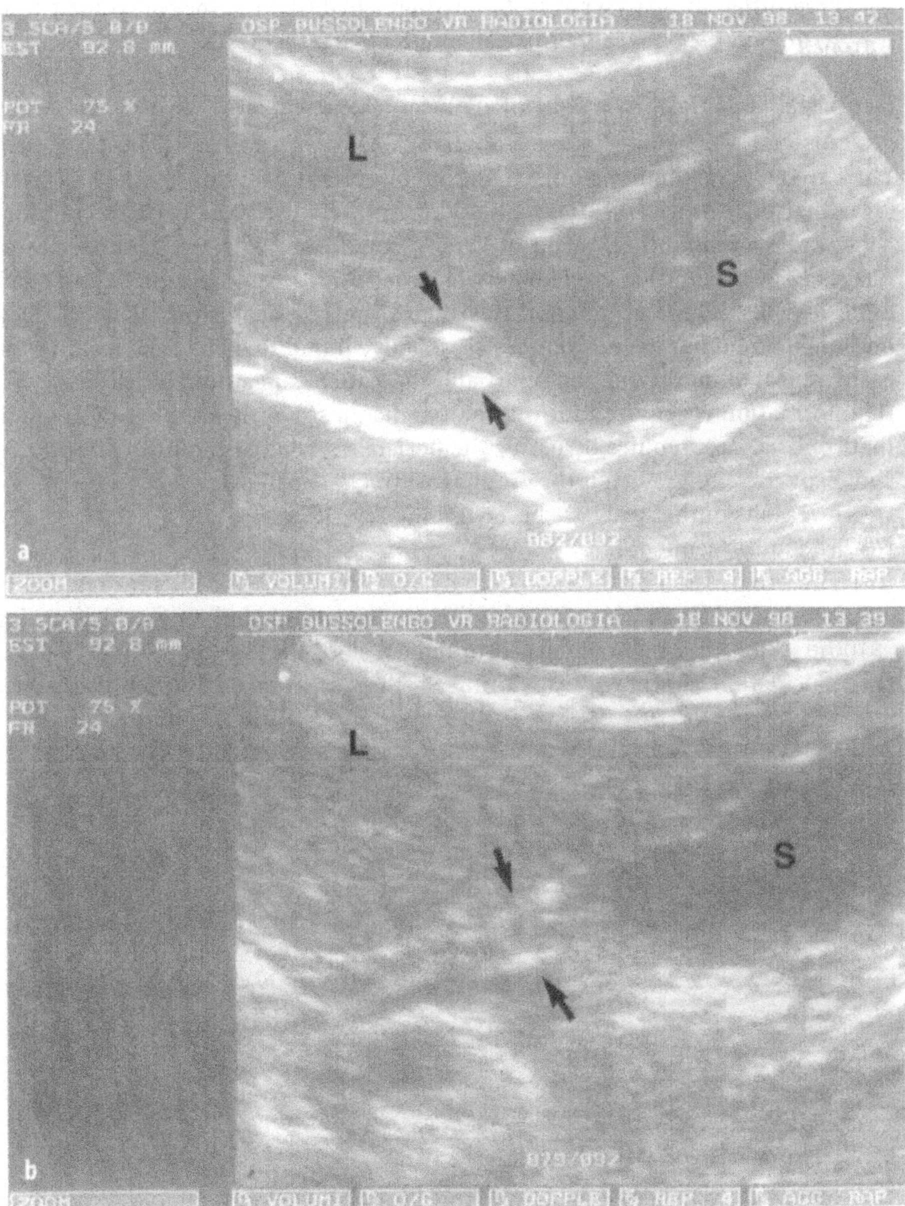

Fig. 2. a Final section of the esophagus (*arrows*) in conditions of normal containment: track-line aspect. **b** Moderate reflux condition with disappearance of track-line aspect owing to advancement of gastric contents in the esophagus (*arrows*). *L*, liver; *S*, stomach

Three different analyses may be distinguished: the esophageal transit test, the physiologic esophageal reflux test and the bile reflux test.

Esophageal Transit Test

The patient, on an empty stomach and in an upright position, is asked to swallow either once or several times a liquid or solid bolus mixed with a nonabsorbable radiocompound (18 MBq of 99mTc colloid or DPTA). A rapid series of images (2 per second) is immediately recorded with a gamma-camera and computer for 30 s. Where esophageal stasis has occurred, acquisition is lengthened once the patient has been given nonradioactive liquid to drink. The test may be easily repeated modifying the bolus and the patient's position. In this way useful information is acquired for differential diagnoses of the esophageal tract, in that solids always require thrust by the peristalsis, whereas liquids can proceed simply by force of gravity, if the esophageal tract is open [4].

The results of the study are based upon:

(ii) The image sequence.

(iii) The progression of the radioactivity-time curves obtained from regions of interest (ROI) at various levels of the esophagus and on the stomach, showing the speed of the bolus and its advancement along the esophageal tract (Fig. 3).

(iii) Calculation of average transit time, of the time it takes to reach the gastric

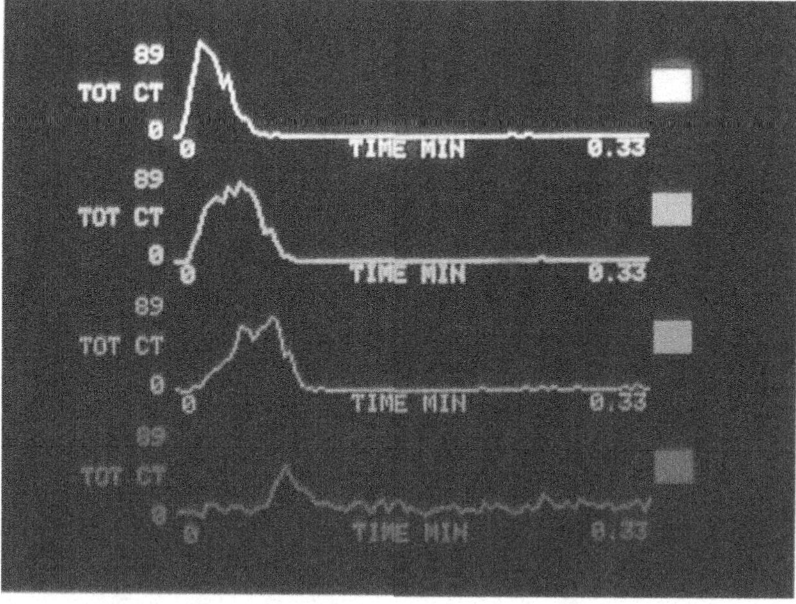

Fig. 3. Esophageal transit test. Radioactivity - time curves on ROI: stomach plus third upper, medium and lower of the esophagus. The gradual appearance over time of the radioactive peak represented by the curves illustrates the advancement of the food bolus along the open esophageal tract, with thrust from the peristaltic wave

cavity, and of residue percentage of the bolus at the level of the esophagus.
(iv) The condensed time-space image, which illustrates two axes in a single functional computerised image: on the vertical axis it shows the advancement of the bolus along the esophagus, and on the horizontal axis it indicates the amount of time which has elapsed (Fig. 4) [5].

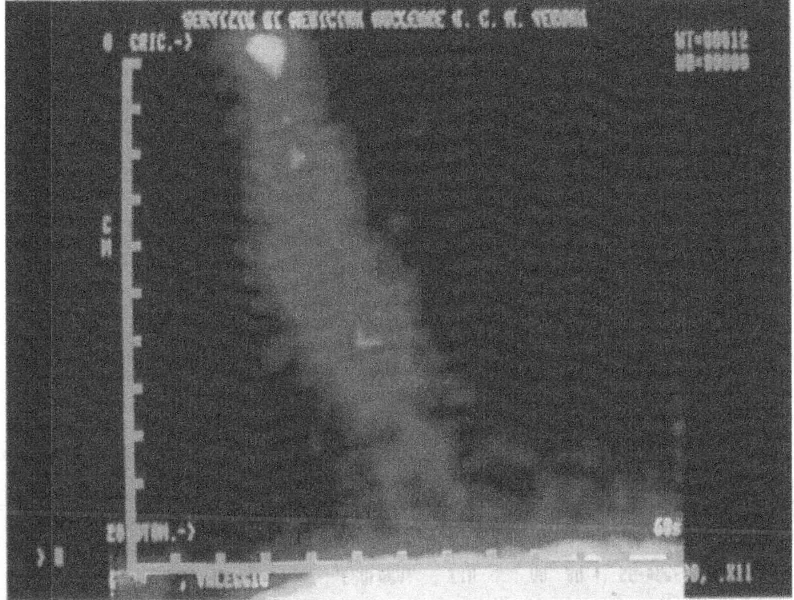

Fig. 4. Esophageal transit test - Condensed image. The functional image shows the regular time-space progression of the radioactive bolus along the esophageal tract, with arrival in the stomach and total emptying of the esophageal area in 5 s

The esophageal transit test documents: delay in the act of swallowing resulting from incoordination; temporary stasis at different levels resulting from slight peristaltic variation or from partial block; intra-esophageal reflux deriving from inverse peristalsis (Fig. 5); gastroesophageal reflux (Fig. 6); any tracer present in the airways during the dynamic stage or when the condition is checked after a period of time has elapsed; total stasis along the entire esophageal tract; and the lengthening of average transit time, of the time it takes to reach the gastric cavity, and of the time it takes for the esophagus to empty.

Motility variations are easily detected in patients with esophagitis from reflux, and are frequently associated with slower transit in organic obstructions. When gastroesophageal reflux occurs, transit time is longer only when there is concomitant variation in esophageal motility [6]. Total stasis of liquids and solids along the entire esophagus is typical of achalasia, whereas in the case of sclerodermata the transit of liquids is less affected [4].

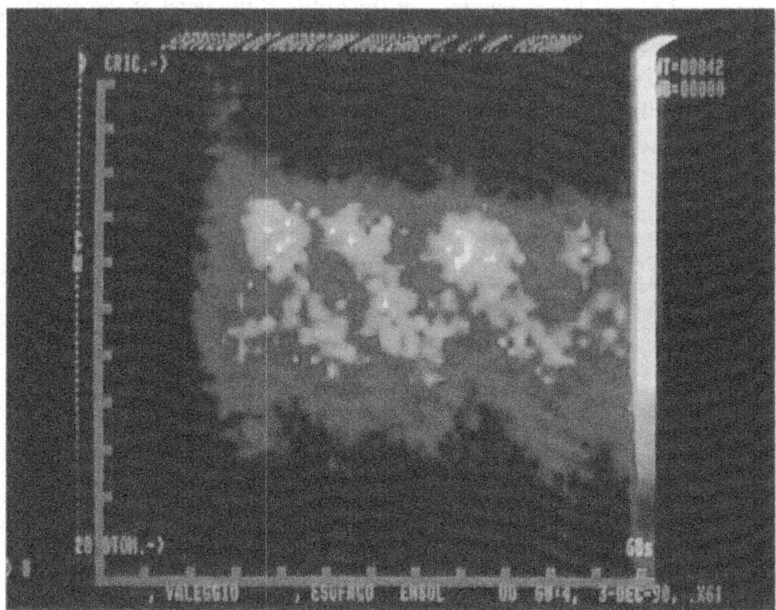

Fig. 5. Intraesophageal reflux from inverse peristalsis. The condensed image shows short repeated stages of progression plus subsequent rising of the solid radioactive bolus to the middle third of the esophagus without reaching the gastric cavity

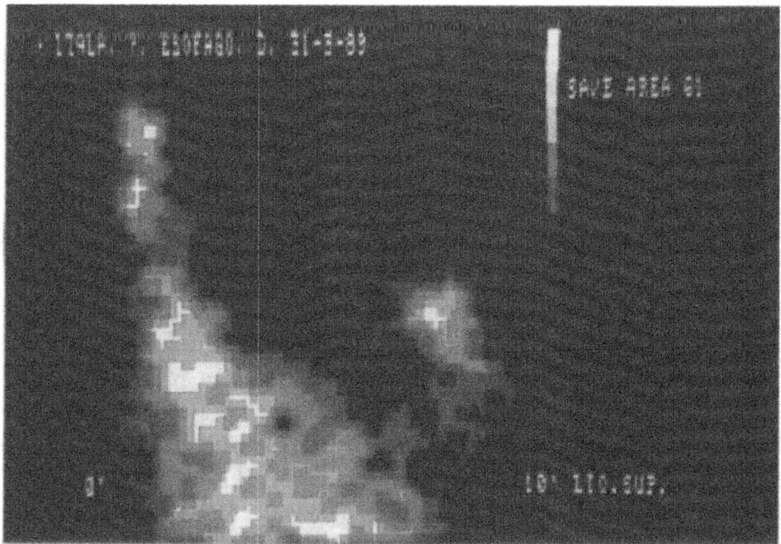

Fig. 6. Gastroesophageal reflux. The condensed image illustrates the regularity of transit in the esophagus with total emptying of the tract in normal time, clearly evidencing the subsequent rising of the radioactive bolus from the stomach to the lower third of the esophagus

Restoring the openness of the esophageal tract normally involves regularising the transit of liquids but not always the transit of solids, owing to persistent peristaltic variations. The test is able to highlight motility variations even in patients reading normal in the dynamic radiological analysis [7].

This test is particularly suitable in patient follow-up on account of its simplicity, its low irradiation dose, and because it offers the possibility of objective quantification of data [8].

Physiological Esophageal Reflux Test

This test may be optionally adopted to illustrate the presence of gastroesophageal reflux in totally physiological conditions. According to the methodology used by Malmud [9], the patient, on an empty stomach from the evening prior to the test, is asked to drink a solution of 150 ml orange juice and 150 ml 0.1 N hydrochloric acid, with 18 MBq of 99mTc nonabsorbable colloid. Once the stomach is filled, a prolonged series of scans is performed, aided by body movements designed to provoke the onset of reflux (increased pressure on the abdomen, Valsava's manoeuvre in the supine position). The registering of reflux in the airways may not be possible until some time has passed (up to 24 h).

The results of the study are based upon:

(i)   Image sequence,

(ii) The progression of radioactive-time curves obtained from the esophagus and the stomach,

(iii) Quantification of the percentage of esophageal radioactivity by comparison with gastric radioactivity (3%-4% when normal).

Reflux is indicated by the presence of radioactivity more or less all the way along the esophageal tract, with a simultaneous rise in the esophageal curve (proportional for height and length to the type and length of the occurrence). The presence of tracer in the airways may be indicated by the presence of spots in the lung area. This test is clinically suited both to the initial diagnosis of reflux, on account of its high degree of sensitivity, and to the monitoring of therapy, in that it is able to quantify the results obtained [8].

Bile Reflux Test

The bile reflux test is an efficient indicator of bile reflux in the esophagus, above all in gastro-resected neoplasia patients, in whom it can provoke ulcerative esophagitis [10].

After an injection of 99m Tc-HIDA (tracer with high hepatocyte concentration and bile elimination) into the vein, the transit of the radiocompound in the intestine is recorded, prolonging the sequential observations for up to 60 min, if necessary with cholecystokinetic stimulus. The aim is to record either the rising of the radiocompound to the level of the gastric stump, or the onset of reflux of radioactive bile in the esophageal tract (Fig. 7). The oral administering of a dose-trace of radiocompound restores the position of esophagus and stomach.

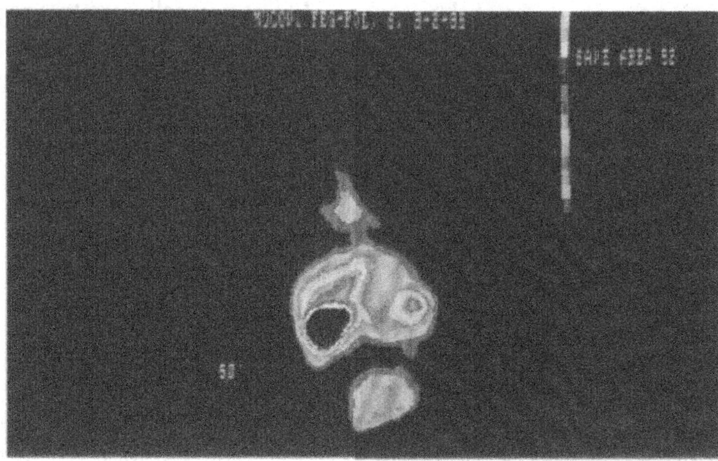

Fig. 7. Esophageal bile reflux. The later stages of the hepatobiliary scintigraph with HIDA highlight not only the normal hepatointestinal transit of the radiocompound, but also the rising back-up of radioactive bile along the esophageal tract

References

1. Gomes H, Menanteau B (1991) Gastroesophageal reflux: comparative study between sonography and pH-monitoring. Pediatr Radiol 21:168-174
2. Di Mario M, Bergami G, Fariello G, Vecchioli Scaldazza A (1995) Diagnosi di reflusso gastroesofageo nell'età pediatrica. Confronto tra ecografia e pasto baritato. Radiol Med 89:76-81
3. Westra SJ, Wolf BHM, Staalman CR (1990) Ultrasound diagnosis of gastroesophageal reflux and hiatal hernia in infants and young children. J Clin Ultrasound 18:477-485
4. Harding LK, Robinson PJA (1991) Gastroenterology. Churchill Livingstone, Edinburgh
5. Svedberg JB (1982) The bolus transport diagram: a functional display method applied to esophageal studies. Clinical Physics and Physiological Measurements 3:267-272
6. Malmud LS, Fischer RS (1982) Scintigraphic evaluation of esophageal transit and gastroesophageal reflux. Semin Nucl Med 12:104-115
7. Malmud LS, Fischer RS (1981) Scintigraphic evaluation of motor function of the upper gastrointestinal tract. Med Clin North Am 65:1291-1310
8. Malmud LS (1986) Radionuclide evaluation of esophageal transit and gastroesophageal reflux. In: Malaguti P, Sciaretta G, Abbati A, Furno A (eds) Radioisotope test in gastroenterology. Masson, Padova, pp 91-97
9. Fisher RS, Malmud LS, Roberts GS, et al (1976) Gastroesophageal (GE) scintiscanning to detect and quantitate GE reflux. Gastroenterology 70:301-308
10. Harding LK, Donovan IA (1986) Bile dynamics. In: Robinson PJ (ed) Nuclear gastroenterology. Churchill Livingstone, Edinburgh, pp 36-51

Further Reading

Tani G, Sciutti R, Teglia F, et al (1993) Diagnosi del reflusso gastroesofageo nell'età pediatrica. Ecografia versus pH-metria. Radiol Med 86:626-629
Wrigth LL, Baker KR, Meny RG (1988) Ultrasound demonstration of gastroesophageal reflux. J Ultrasound Med 7:471-475

The Esophageal Scintiscan

M. Gasparini, A. Bruno, and P. Gerundini

Introduction

Despite advances in medical imaging techniques, such as computed tomography, ultrasound and magnetic resonance, nuclear medicine remains a growing speciality. The clinical practice of nuclear medicine is based on the use of radioactive materials (radionuclides) for the purposes of diagnosis and therapy. This technique is noninvasive and safe; in the majority of cases the administration of diagnostic doses of radiolabeled tracers results in no more radiation exposure than X-ray procedures. The behaviour of a biological substance of interest may be studied by introducing a small quantity of the tracer in a suitably radiolabeled form. The introduction of the tracer should not affect the behaviour of the substance under investigation, there must be stable attachment of the radiolabel to the parent molecule, and the radiolabel should be easily and accurately detected.

In nuclear medicine, the most important and widely utilized radionuclide is the technetium-99m (^{99m}Tc). In fact, this radionuclide has many advantages, including a higher photon energy (140 KeV) which is optimal for gamma camera imaging. The short physical half-life (6 h) permits a larger dose to be administered. Furthermore, ^{99m}Tc can be produced on site by a generator, which makes it readily available and relatively inexpensive. Radionuclide imaging studies of gastrointestinal tract are generally far less invasive than the alternative X-ray contrast procedure. It is possible to use more physiological tracers, which adds to the clinical value in both diagnosis and research.

The evaluation of esophageal motor disorders often requires the use of multiple diagnostic modalities. Each method has certain advantages and disadvantages. Barium radiography is useful for excluding structural lesions of the esophagus and detecting mucosal changes. Cinefluorography provides qualitative but not quantitative information about function. Endoscopy is also commonly used to detect structural and mucosal changes, but is of no value in diag-

Nuclear Medicine Department, IRCCS Ospedale Maggiore, Milan, Italy

nosing disorders of motility. Esophageal manometry provides useful information on the amplitude, duration, and velocity of peristaltic contractions, on sphincter pressure and on the ability of the upper esophageal sphincter (UES) and lower esophageal sphincter (LES) to relax. It is the standard procedure for making a definitive diagnosis of esophageal motility disorders; specific manometric criteria exist for each entity. Since manometry requires passing a catheter through the nose or mouth, patients are often not keen on undergoing this procedure.

Radionuclide Esophageal Transit

In 1972 Kazem [1] first described the use of radionuclides to evaluate esophageal transit. Since then, many variations on this technique have been developed, for example with respect to the radionuclide used, the bolus content, patient positioning, and the method of acquisition (Table 1). A general protocol for esophageal transit studies could be described as follows: practice swallows are performed in the supine position; then 5.55-18.5 MBq of ^{99m}Tc sulfur colloid (^{99m}Tc-SC) in 10-15 ml water is swallowed as a bolus. Dynamic images are acquired (0.1-0.8 frames/s) on a computer. Dry swallows follow at defined intervals (e.g. 30 s). The individual images and cinematic display are reviewed. Regions of interest can be drawn on the computer and time-activity curves can be generated. Quantification may be performed (transit time or percent clearance) and functional images (e.g. condensed dynamic images) can be constructed and reviewed.

Table 1. Methodologies for performing esophageal transit studies. (Modified from [52])

Author	Bolus	Dose	Position	Acquisition	Quantification
Kazem [1]	Tc-O$_4$	0.5-1.0 mCi in 10-20 ml tea	Erect	0.4 s/frame for 1.0-1.5 min	Time/activity curves
Tolin et al. [6]	Tc-SC	150 µCi in 15 ml H$_2$O	Supine	1 s/frame for 15 min, then 15 s/ frame for 10 min	% Emptying
Russel et al. [9]	Tc-SC	250 µCi in 10 ml H$_2$O	Supine	0.4 s/frame for 50 s	Transit time
Tatsch et al. [3]	Tc-SC	250 µCi in 10 ml H$_2$O	Supine	0.8 s/frame for 240 s	Transit time Condensed images
Drane et al. [22]	Tc-SC	100-300 µCi	Supine	0.5 s/frame for 50 s	Transit time % Emptying

$Tc\text{-}O_4^-$, pertechnetate; $Tc\text{-}SC$, sulfur colloid radiolabeled with Tc-O$_4$

^{99m}Tc-SC in water is the most commonly used radiopharmaceutical for esophageal transit studies; it is inexpensive, easy to prepare, neither absorbed nor secreted by the esophageal mucosa, and has optimal physical characteristics for imaging. An alternative is Krypton-81m in solution, eluted from a Rb-81/Kr generator [2]. This has the advantage of a high count rate and a minimal absorbed radiation dose because of its 13-s half-life, but it is expensive and not widely available.

A swallowed liquid bolus, usually water, is most commonly used to evaluate esophageal transit. However, semi-solid boluses of jam, gelatin, hamburger, chelex resin in oatmeal, cold cereal with milk, and others are also used. Recent reports suggest that semisolid boluses may be more sensitive than liquids for detecting abnormal esophageal transit [3-5]. The supine position is usually recommended because it eliminates the effect of gravity on esophageal emptying [6]. However, the upright position may help to distinguish achalasia (in which the LES does not relax) from systemic sclerosis (with a hypotensive LES), since a liquid bolus may not empty from the esophagus in achalasia in the supine position.

The radiation dose absorbed by patients from radionuclide esophageal transit studies is low (Table 2), particularly when compared to that received from fluoroscopy and cine-esophagography.

Consistency, position, and volume all influence normal esophageal transit. Transit is faster for liquids than for more viscous materials, with the patient upright compared to supine, and for smaller (10 ml) compared to larger volumes (20 ml). Multiple swallows are often required even in healthy subjects to

Table 2. Absorbed radiation from 37 MBq ^{99m}Tc-SC gastroesophageal scintigraphy, by age group. (Modified from [53])

Organ	Absorbed dose (cGy)				
	Newborn	1 year	5 years	10 years	Adult
Stomach	0.383	0.093	0.050	0.031	0.018
ULI	0.569	0.267	0.164	0.090	0.052
LLI	0.927	0.380	0.194	0.120	0.033
Ovaries	0.099	0.042	0.033	0.072	0.010
Testes	0.018	0.007	0.003	0.011	0.000
Thyroid	0.002	0.0006	0.0002	0.0001	0.000
TB	0.020	0.011	0.006	0.004	0.002

ULI, upper large intestine; *LLI*, lower large intestine; *TB*, total body

completely empty the esophagus. A high incidence of "aberrant" swallows (up to 25%) has been observed in normal people [7, 8]. Valid quantitative analysis requires that the patient swallow the tracer bolus in one go; pharyngeal time-activity curves may help establish that this has occurred [9].

The esophageal transit time is defined as the time from initial entry of the bolus into the esophagus until total clearance from the esophagus. Patients with achalasia, diffuse spasm, scleroderma, aperistalsis associated with diabetes, and nonspecific motor disorders have transit times longer than 15 s (normal mean, 7 ± 3 s). Patients with achalasia often have transit times longer than 50 s, which limits the method's ability to estimate the severity of disease (Fig. 1).

Normal mean liquid esophageal transit times vary slightly depending on the technique used, but are usually in the range of 6-10 s, with an accepted upper normal range of 10-15 s [9-12]. Several kinds of pattern analyses based on computer-generated curves or functional images have been used as aids to diagnosis.

Functional images have been found useful by several investigators [2, 10, 13]. As an alternative to viewing the many images acquired in a single transit study, the dynamic data can be condensed into a single image (condensed dynamic images, CDIs) with one spatial dimension (vertical) and one temporal dimension (horizontal). The technique is based on the fact that one is interested only in craniocaudal transit, not lateral motion.

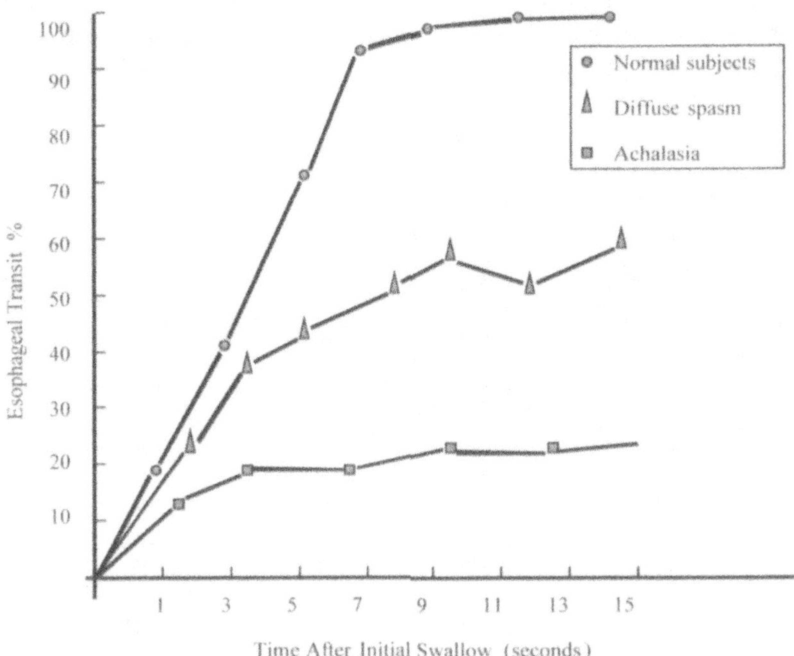

Fig. 1. Mean esophageal transit time-activity curves after a single swallow in 15 normal subjects, 8 patients with achalasia and 10 patients with diffuse esophageal spasm

Findings in Esophageal Motility Disorders

Achalasia is characterized by the absence of peristalsis in the distal two-thirds of the esophagus, increased LES pressure, and incomplete relaxation with swallowing. The result is esophageal dilatation and retention of food. Patients complain of dysphagia with both liquids and solids, weight loss, noctural regurgitation, cough, and occasional aspiration. The etiology is unknown. A barium swallow shows esophageal dilatation with smooth tapering at the gastroesophageal junction. Tumors can be excluded by endoscopy. The diagnosis of achalasia is confirmed by manometry, which shows aperistalsis and incomplete LES relaxation. Elevated LES pressure is common. Radionuclide esophageal transit studies are very sensitive (93%-100%) and can be used to reach a diagnosis in a noninvasive manner [6, 9, 14, 15].

Diffuse esophageal spasm is characterized by intermittent chest pain or dysphagia without a demonstrable organic lesion. The symptoms are produced by abnormal nonperistaltic contractions of the esophageal body, which can be demonstrated by manometry or radiological studies. Specific manometric criteria are required to make this diagnosis [18]; radionuclide transit studies have a moderate sensitivity (67%-77%) for detecting this condition [17].

The "nutcracker esophagus" is a somewhat controversial diagnosis [18, 19]. These patients typically have noncardiac chest pain and normal radiographic findings. High-amplitude peristaltic contractions, sometimes of prolonged duration, are found at manometry [20]. The sensitivity of radionuclide transit studies for this condition ranges from 0% to 94% [21, 22].

Nonspecific motor disorder is a diagnosis used in patients who have abnormal manometry but do not fit into other well-defined categories. The sensitivity of radionuclide transit studies for detecting this entity is variable (42%-100%) [23].

Scleroderma, a systemic disease involving the smooth muscle of the esophagus, often shows aperistalsis, a dilated esophagus, and retention of barium and gastroesophageal reflux (GER) on barium radiographs. Manometry may demonstrate decreased or absent LES pressure and decreased amplitude of peristaltic contractions, or aperistalsis confined to the smooth muscle portion of the esophagus. Radionuclide transit studies have found delayed emptying [24]. Systemic lupus erythematosus and polymyositis may also be associated with smooth muscle disease of the esophagus and abnormal esophageal transit studies [25]. Striated muscle abnormalities of muscular dystrophy, myasthenia gravis, dermatomyositis/polymyositis, and myotonic dystrophy can cause loss of propulsive force in the pharyngeal muscles and impairment of the coordinated transfer of food from pharynx to esophagus, manifested by difficulty in initiating the act of swallowing. Radionuclide transit studies may detect abnormalities in these patients [26].

Diabetes and alcoholism are often associated with abnormalities of esophageal motor function. In diabetics, this is associated with gastroenteropathy [27]. Esophageal motility disorders have also been described with GER and esophagitis.

Symptomatic reflux of gastric contents into the esophagus is one of the most common gastrointestinal disorders. Gastroesophageal reflux disease (GERD) refers to a symptomatic clinical condition and/or the histological changes that result from episodes of GER, while reflux esophagitis refers to the mucosal changes of inflammation, hyperplasia, and erosions that often occur secondary to GER. Only 30%-40% of patients with heartburn have mucosal injury. Heartburn is the most common clinical complaint. Other symptoms include chest pain, regurgitation, and sour breath. Regurgitation and aspiration may cause respiratory symptoms of asthma and recurrent pneumonia. Other serious complications of GERD include stricture, bleeding, and perforation. Dysphagia is usually a symptom of stricture. In some patients a peculiar reparative process occurs, whereby squamous epithelium of the esophagus is replaced by metaplastic columnar-type epithelium, known as Barrett's esophagus. This entity is important because it is associated with a 10% incidence of adenocarcinoma. The symptoms of GER in infants and children differ considerably from those in adults. In addition to excessive regurgitation, the predominant symptoms are respiratory distress, iron deficiency anemia, and failure to thrive.

A variety of tests have been used to diagnose GERD. Barium esophagography can detect severe grades of reflux, mucosal damage, strictures, and tumors; however, it has a low overall sensitivity for detecting GERD. This is not surprising because the morphological changes of esophagitis are difficult to detect even at endoscopy without the benefit of biopsy. Endoscopy is commonly used, provides a direct view of the esophageal mucosa, and allows biopsy. The Bernstein acid infusion test attempts to reproduce the patient's symptoms and confirm their esophageal origin by infusing 0.1 N hydrochloric acid into the distal esophagus. Esophageal manometry allows quantitative assessment of esophageal body motor function in response to swallowing and acid infusion.

The Tuttle acid reflux test requires that a pH electrode be positioned in the distal esophagus 5 cm above the LES. An abrupt drop of the esophageal pH to less than 4.0 is associated with GER. Proper placement is a critical factor in the correct interpretation of this test. This study is performed during basal conditions and after acid loading. Although false-negatives and false-positives do occur, it is generally considered the gold standard for the diagnosis of GER.

A test that is increasingly used is extended (12 to 24-hour) pH monitoring. It is typically performed in symptomatic patients without evidence of esophagitis by esophagography or endoscopy. Continuous pH monitoring is now possible while the patient continues normal daily activities.

Radionuclide GER scintigraphy has a number of potential advantages over the other diagnostic procedures discussed. It is more physiological, easily performed, well tolerated by the patient, and quantitative. The radiation exposure is considerably lower than that associated with other radiographic procedures commonly used to evaluate the esophagus. Although its sensitivity has been reported to be as high as 90%, some studies have found it to be considerably lower, 14%-78% [28-30]. Some recent reviews of GER do not even mention it as a diagnostic option, describe radionuclide methods as "obsolete and replaced by pH monitoring" [31], reserve its role for a subgroup of selected patients (e.g. those with alkaline reflux or atrophic gastritis), or use it solely for investigational purposes. An important reason for this seems to be the existence of many competing modalities performed by gastroenterologists. In contrast, pediatricians seem to believe that scintigraphy is very useful for evaluating GER in children [32, 33]. It is interesting to note that the accuracy in adults and children appears to be quite similar, with a sensitivity between 57% and 88% [30, 34].

Much of the original investigation and validation of adult GER scintigraphy was performed at Temple University. Several reviews have updated their results. Initially, they studied 30 patients with symptoms of GER and a positive acid-reflux test. Scintigraphy was found to have a sensitivity of 90% for detecting GER, which was better than that of other methods including hiatal hernia seen on radiography (60%), fluoroscopic reflux (50%), LES pressure < 15 mm Hg (77%), acid perfusion test (63%), histological esophagitis (47%) and endoscopic esophagitis (40%). At present over 1000 patients have been studied and an overall sensitivity of 88%-91% has been reported [35, 36].

Kaul et al. [37] studied 69 adults with GER symptoms and endoscopic esophagitis. The sensitivity of scintigraphy was 86%, significantly higher than that of intraesophageal pH measurements (70%) and contrast esophagography (28%). The severity of esophagitis correlated with positive GER scintigraphy. By contrast, Hoffman and Vansant [38], using a similar method, identified GER in only 4 of 29 patients who showed other evidence of reflux by either fluoroscopically monitored barium swallow, esophagogastroscopy, or esophageal biopsy. Interestingly, the pH reflux study had a similar low sensitivity. They concluded that both tests were too insensitive to be of value in the diagnosis of GERD.

In an interesting study, Shay et al. [39] performed simultaneous pH monitoring and continuous scintigraphy (5-frames) for 40 min in 9 patients with histologically proven severe reflux esophagitis. Scintigraphy detected 61% of all events as opposed to 16% for pH monitoring. The two techniques detected the same events in only 23% of 218 reflux events. GER scintigraphy detected more reflux events during the first 20 min, and pH monitoring detected more events during the second 20 min. However, when scintigraphy was compared to short-term pH probe monitoring, considered to be the gold standard, it was shown to be quite sensitive, certainly more sensitive than the only other technique that directly measures reflux, i.e. radiography with fluoroscopy. The poor results obtained in some studies [38] distort the overall results. The reasons for this are unclear, although in one of these studies pH monitoring had a similar low sensitivity.

Radionuclide GER studies play a much more important clinical role in pediatrics. This is probably due to pediatricians' preferences for noninvasive procedures and the difficulties involved in performing invasive and technically demanding studies in children.

Pediatric GER is most common in infants 6-9 months of age. It usually becomes apparent by the age of 2 months but in the majority of cases it is self-limited, resolving spontaneously by the end of infancy. Approximately one-third of the patients have persistent symptoms until the age of four. GER has been implicated as a cause of recurrent respiratory infections, asthma, failure to thrive, esophagitis, esophageal stricture, chronic blood loss, and the sudden infant death syndrome. Symptoms and signs of GER in children include chronic nocturnal cough, poor weight gain, vomiting, aspiration or choking, asthmatic episodes, stridor, and apnea. As in adults, a variety of diagnostic methods have been used, with the 24-hour pH probe being the gold standard.

The radionuclide method involves feeding the infant a meal that approximates its normal feed, usually formula or milk, although juice has also been used, with 4-40 MBq ^{99m}Tc-SC as the radiolabel. A concentration of 200 kBq/ml has been recommended for optimum imaging [30]. After the infant has burped, it is placed in the supine position with the scintillation camera positioned either anteriorly or posteriorly [40] and the chest and upper abdomen in the field of view. Abdominal compression is not normally used because it is considered nonphysiological; it is poorly tolerated in infants and there is evidence that it does not increase the detection rate for reflux. Data is acquired on a computer and the study lasts 60-120 min [48]. An acquisition time of 60 min has been shown to increase the detection rate for GER by 25% compared to 30 min. Reflux events are graded by level (low or high), duration (e.g. more or less than 10 s), and by their temporal relationship to food intake. Longer reflux events increase the risk of esophagitis; events with smaller gastric volumes may have more clinical significance because the reflux occurs without the increased pressure of a full meal volume and a lack of acid buffering. Evidence of pulmonary aspiration is sought in the dynamic study but infrequently found. For maximum sensitivity, static high count images are obtained at 1 and 2-4 hours, and sometimes also the next morning

An esophageal transit study can be performed either before or after the reflux study. In addition to diagnosing an associated motility disorder, a "salivagram" may often detect pulmonary aspiration when the GER study is negative [41].

Heyman et al. [30] reported a new scintigraphic technique for detecting GER in a study involving 48 children. After intake of a normal milk feed with ^{99m}Tc, images were obtained on a computer at a rate of 1 frame/min for 60 min. Computer processing and calculation of GER and gastric emptying were performed. Radiographic studies were available for comparison in 39 patients. There was agreement in 20 patients, both showing reflux in 7 (18%) and no reflux in 13 cases (33%). The radionuclide study was positive in 59%; barium radiography was positive in 26%.

Blumhagen et al. [42] used the acid reflux test as the standard for evaluating 65 infants and children with GER scintigraphy. After ingestion of labeled apple juice, images were acquired continuously (30 s/frame) for 30-60 min. The overall sensitivity for GER was 75% and the specificity was 71%.

In summary, there is general agreement that GER scintigraphy is a valuable and clinically useful technique for pediatric patients. Rapid acquisition methods are more sensitive; however, the exact cutoff between normal and abnormal in infants is uncertain. Increased significance should be assigned to frequent and high-level GER, reflux as the stomach contents diminish, and associated delayed clearance or a motility disorder. A radionuclide transit study performed as part of the same study can both evaluate motility and detect aspiration with high sensitivity.

All images of the dynamic GER study should be reviewed. Cine-display is often helpful. Time-activity curves can be generated from regions of interest drawn for the oropharynx, esophagus, and stomach. GER is seen as distinct spikes of activity into the esophagus. The time-activity curves should be evaluated in conjunction with the images because patient movement may result in gastric activity appearing in the esophageal region. Some do not consider episodes of GER in the first 5 min to be abnormal unless prolonged [43, 44], while others believe that all episodes are abnormal.

A variety of quantitative indices used in adult populations may also be useful for pediatric studies. From the mean value of the esophageal time-activity curve evaluated as a percentage of the initial gastric activity of Devos et al. [45] to the derived reflux index obtained by integrating the esophageal time-activity curve over 60 min and dividing this by the initial gastric activity of Heyman et al. [34], Piepsz et al. [46] determined the percent activity in an episode relative to the gastric activity at that time, multiplied by the duration of the episode in multiples of 20 s. The resulting values were added up for the 60-minute study. Peaks greater than 5% generally corresponded to reflux.

Delayed images are routinely obtained for evidence of pulmonary aspiration. Best results require high-count delayed images 2-4 hours after feeding. Although some have suggested to acquire morning images after an evening meal, the radiolabeled aspirated meal may clear due to its relatively short residence time in the lung. Several authors have concluded that overnight images add little additional information [47]. Most studies have shown a relatively low detection rate for the 2 to 4-hour delayed images. The salivagram seems a better indicator of pulmonary aspiration [41].

Aspiration pneumonia is one of the most serious complications of gastrostomy tube feeding, with a reported incidence of 10%-20% in nursing home patients. An interesting prospective study was performed by Coben and coworkers [48] in 10 patients in whom they examined LES pressure before and after placement of gastrostomy tubes. The authors evaluated the effects of rapid intragastric bolus and slow, continuous feeding on LES pressure. All patients were evaluated with scintigrams obtained after a rapid bolus infusion of 250 ml Jevity (a particular mixture of proteins, carbohydrates and fat with a fixed osmolality), labeled with 192 MBq ^{99m}Tc sulfur colloid. Scintigrams were obtained to determine GER every 10 s over a 15-minute period. The examination was repeated after 24 hours. The authors concluded that rapid intragastric bolus feeding via the gastrostomy tube causes transient relaxation of the LES, and suggested to modify the procedure by which patients are fed via gastrostomy tubes so that the risk of aspiration pneumonia can be diminished.

Another important condition in which nuclear medicine can play an important diagnostic role is Zenker's diverticulum, which is an outpouching of the esophageal wall in the natural weakness of the posterior hypopharyngeal wall.

Surgical treatment is indicated to relieve symptoms such as dysphagia and regurgitation, and to prevent aspiration pneumonia. Standard surgery includes cricopharyngeal myotomy and diverticulectomy or suspension of the diverticulum through a left cervicotomy. The endoscopic approach consists of the division of the septum between the pouch and the cervical esophagus, thus establishing a common cavity with simultaneous section of the UES [49].

Our group at the Ospedale Maggiore of Milan studied the effectiveness of this new technique in the treatment of Zenker's diverticulum by means of radionuclide pharyngoesophageal transit in addition to clinical and manometric evaluation [50, 51]. Ninty-five patients underwent a transoral stapled diverticulum esophagostomy. None of these patients had had previous endoscopic or surgical treatment for their disorder. All patients complained of dysphagia and pharyngo-oral regurgitation and 18 patients had a history of recurrent respiratory infections most likely resulting from aspiration. Esophageal scintigraphy was performed in the upright position after a single swallow of 15 ml water containing 18-37 MBq ^{99m}Tc sulfur colloid.

After data acquistion, time-activity curves were generated by drawing regions of interest using dedicated software. The following parameters were derived from the upper esophageal time-activity curve: the time necessary to clear 50% and 75% (T50 and T75) of the maximum activity recorded in the upper esophageal region of interest and the percentage of the maximum activity remaining in the upper esophagus at 1 and 10 min (R1 and R10). The severity of the symptoms of dysphagia was scored before and after surgery as follows: 0 (absent); 1 (mild) occasional; 2 (moderate) daily symptoms requiring liquid to clear; and 3 (severe) requiring liquid diet for symptoms. The scoring for regurgitation was performed as follows: 0 (absent); 1 (mild) occasional symptoms; 2 (moderate), daily symptoms; and 3 (severe) respiratory symptoms and/or complications.

The preoperative workup included standard barium esophagogram, upper gastrointestinal endoscopy, and esophageal manometry. The median size of the diverticulum measured by flexible endoscopy was 4.0 cm (range, 2.5-8 cm). At a mean follow-up of 23 months (range, 13-48 months) the mean dysphagia score decreased from 2.6 ± 0.5 to 0.8 ± 0.5 ($p < 0.001$) and the mean regurgitation score decreased from 2.6 ± 1.0 to 0.3 ± 0.5 ($p < 0.05$). Upper esophageal sphincter resting decreased from 52.4 ± 25.8 to 31.5 ± 12.2 mm Hg ($p < 0.001$).

This study shows that transoral diverticulum-esophagostomy relieves symptoms and decreases outflow resistance at the pharyngoesophageal junction. The division of the common wall by stapling is an innovative procedure that appears to be simpler and safer than electrocoagulation or laser. In Fig. 2 an example of Zenker's diverticulum before and after surgery is reported. Compared with conventional surgery the advantages of the endosurgical approach include absence of skin incision, shorter operation time and shorter hospital stay. This study demonstrates the utility also in minimally invasive transoral stapled diverticulum esophagostomy in patients with Zenker's diverticulum.

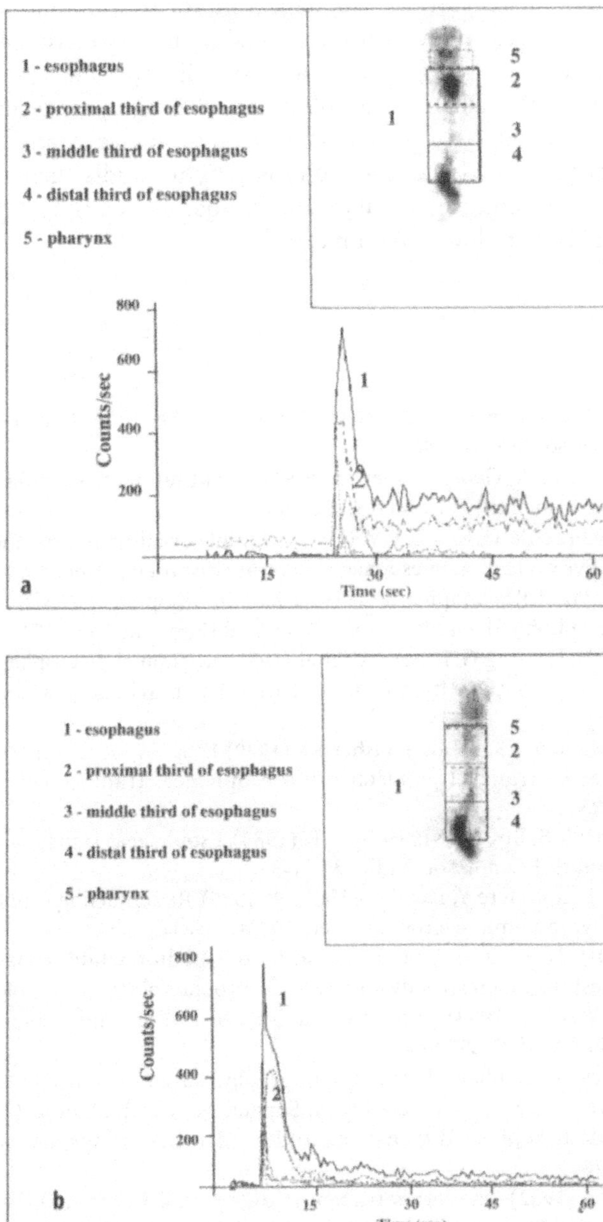

Fig. 2a,b. Esophageal transit in a patient with Zenker's diverticulum before (**a**) and after (**b**) diverticulum esophagostomy

Conclusions

Functional symptoms caused by esophageal motor dysfunction are relatively common in the general population. Knowledge of the relationship between symptoms and the underlying esophageal dysmotility provides physicians with a basis for successful evaluation and treatment. Scintigraphic techniques allow noninvasive and quantitative assessment of physiological transit throughout the gastrointestinal tract. In contrast to radiographic studies using barium and manometric studies requiring nasal or oral intubation, scintigraphy is noninvasive and associated with low radiation exposure.

References

1. Kazem I (1972) A new scintigraphic technique for the study of the esophagus. AJR Am J Roentgenol 115:681-688
2. Ham HR, Piepsz A, Georges B, et al (1984) Quantitation of esophageal transit by means of Kr-81m. Eur J Nucl Med 9:362-365
3. Tatsch K, Schroettle U, Kirsch CM (1991) Multiple swallow test for the quantitative and qualitative evaluation of esophageal motility disorders. J Nucl Med 32:1365-1370
4. Steffey DL, Wahl RL, Shapiro B (1986) Diabetic oesophagoparesis: assessment by solid phase radionuclide scintigraphy. Nucl Med Commun 7:165-171
5. Holloway RH, Krosing G, Lange RC, et al (1983) Radionuclide esophageal emptying of a solid meal to quantitate results of therapy in achalasia. Gastroenterology 84:771-776
6. Tolin RD, Malmud LS, Reilly J, Fisher RS (1979) Esophageal scintigraphy to quantitate esophageal transit (quantitation of esophageal transit). Gastroenterology 76:1402-1408
7. Styles CB, Holt S, Bowles KL, Hopper R (1984) Esophageal transit scintigraphy - a cautionary note. J Can Assoc Radiol 35:31-33
8. Carrette S, Lacourciere Y, Lavoie S, Halle P (1985) Radionuclide esophageal transit in progressive systemic sclerosis. J Rheum 12:478-481
9. Russell COH, Hill LD, Holmes ER, et al (1981) Radionuclide transit: a sensitive screening test for esophageal dysfunction. Gastroenterology 80:887-892
10. Klein HA, Wald A (1984) Computer analysis of radionuclide esophageal transit studies. J Nucl Med 25:957-964
11. Klein HA (1995) Esophageal transit scintigraphy. Semin Nucl Med 4:306-317
12. Lamas-Elvira JM, Martinez-Peredes M, Sopena-Monforte M, et al (1986) Value of radionuclide oesophageal transit in studies of function dysphagia. Br J Radiol 59:1073-1078
13. Svedberg JB (1982) The bolus transport diagram: a functional display method applied to oesophageal studies. Clin Phys Physiol Meas 3:267-272
14. Rozen P, Gelfond M, Zaltaman, S, Baron J, Gilat T (1982) Dynamic, diagnostic, and pharmacological radionuclide studies of the esophagus in achalasia. Radiology 144:587-590
15. DeCaesteker JS, Blackwell JN, Adam RD, et al (1986) Clinical value of radionuclide esophageal transit measurement. Gut 27:659-666
16. Richter JE, Castell DO (1984) Diffuse esophageal spasm: a reappraisal. Ann Intern Med 100:242-245

17. Blackwell J, Haanan WWJ, Adam RD, Heading RC (1984) Radionuclide transit studies in the detection of oesophageal dysmotility. Gut 24:421-426
18. Richter JE, Wu WC, Cowan RJ, Ott DJ, Blackwell JN (1987) Letter to the editor: nutcracker esophagus. Dig Dis Sci 30:188-190
19. Richter JE, Wu WC, Ott DJ, Chen YM (1987) "Nutcracker" esophagus: diagnosis with radionuclide esophageal scintigraphy versus manometry. Radiology 164:877-879 (letter)
20. Benjamin SB, Gerhardt DC, Castell DO (1979) High amplitude, peristaltic esophageal contractions associated with chest pain and/or dysphagia. Gastroenterology 77:478-483
21. Richter JE, Blackwell JN, Wu WC, et al (1987) Relationship of radionuclide liquid bolus transport and esophageal manometry. J Lab Clin Med 109:217-224
22. Drane WE, Johnson DA, Hagan DP, Cattau EL (1987) "Nutcracker" esophagus: diagnosis with radionuclide esophageal scintigraphy versus manometry. Radiology 163:33-37
23. Mughal MM, Marples M, Bancewicz J (1986) Scintigraphic assessment of esophageal motility: what does it show and how reliable is it? Gut 27:946-953
24. Drane WE, Karvelis K, Johnson DA, et al (1986) Progressive systemic sclerosis: radionuclide esophageal scintigraphy and manometry. Radiology 160:73-76
25. Horowitz M, McNeil JD, Maddern JG, et al (1986) Abnormalities of gastric and esophageal emptying in polymyositis and dermatomyositis. Gastroenterology 90:434-439
26. Eckern VF, Nix W, Kraus W, Bohl J (1986) Esophageal motor function in patients with muscular dystrophy. Gastroenterology 90:628-630
27. Russel COH, Gannan FR, Coatsworth J, et al (1983) Relationship among esophageal dysfunction, diabetic gastroenteropathy and peripheral neuropathy. Dig Dis Sci 28:289-293
28. Fisher RS, Malmud LS, Roberts GS, Lobis IF (1976) Gastroesophageal (GE) scintiscanning to detect and quantitate GE reflux. Gastroenterology 70:301-308
29. Velasco N, Pope CE, Gannan RM, et al (1984) Measurement of esophageal reflux by scintigraphy. Dig Dis Sci 11:977-982
30. Heyman S, Kirkpatrick, JA, Winter HS, Treves S (1979) An improved radionuclide method for the diagnosis of gastroesophageal reflux and aspiration in children (milk scan). Radiology 131:479-482
31. Wu WC (1990) Ancillary test in the diagnosis of gastroesophageal reflux disease. In: McCallum RW, Mittal RK (eds) Gastroenterology clinics of North America, vol. 19. WB Saunders, Philadelphia, pp 671-682
32. Dalla Vecchia LK, Grosfeld JL, West KW, et al (1997) Reoperation after Nissen fundoplication in children with gastroesophageal reflux. Experience with 130 patients. Ann Surg 226:315-323
33. Sondheimer JM (1988) Gastroesophageal reflux: update on pathogenesis and diagnosis. Pediatr Clin N Am 35:103-153
34. Arasu TS, Wyllie R, Fitzgerald JF, et al (1980) Gastroesophageal reflux in infants and children: comparative accuracy of diagnostic methods. J Pediatr 96:798-803
35. Malmud LS, Fisher RS (1988) Scintigraphic evaluation of esophageal transit, gastroesophageal reflux, and gastric emptying. In: Gottschalk A, Hoffer PB, Potchen EJ (eds) Diagnostic nuclear medicine, 2nd edn. Williams & Wilkins, Baltimore, pp 663-683
36. Fisher RS, Malmud LS (1980) Functional scintigraphy: diagnostic applications in gastroenterology. In: Berk JE (ed) Developments in digestive disease. Lea & Febiger, Philadelphia, pp 139-164
37. Kaul B, Petersen H, Grette K, Erichsen H, Myrvold HE (1985) Scintigraphy, pH mea-

surement, and radiography in the evaluation of gastroesophageal reflux. Scand J Gastroenterol 20:289-294

38. Hoffman GC, Vansant JH (1979) The gastroesophageal scintiscan. Arch Surg 114:727-728

39. Shay SS, Eggli D, Johnson L (1991) Simultaneous esophageal pH monitoring and scintigraphy during the postprandial period in patients with severe reflux esophagitis. Dig Dis Sci 36:558-564

40. Rosen P, Treves ST (1985) Gastroesophageal reflux and gastric emptying. In: Treves ST (ed) Pediatric nuclear medicine. Springer, Berlin Heidelberg New York, pp 171-177

41. Heyman S, Respondek M (1989) Detection of pulmonary aspiration in children by radionuclide salivagram. J Nucl Med 30:697-699

42. Blumhagen JD, Rudd TG, Christie DL (1980) Gastroesophageal reflux in children: radionuclide gastroesophagography. AJR Am J Roentgenol 135:1001-1004

43. Heyman S (1985) Pediatric nuclear gastroenterology: evaluation of gastroesophageal reflux and gastrointestinal bleeding. In: Freeman LM, Weissmann HS (eds) Nuclear medicine annual 1985. Raven, New York, pp 33-53

44. Piepsz A, Georges B, Rodeschj P, Cadranel S (1982) Gastroesophageal scintiscanning in children. J Nucl Med 23: 631-632

45. Devos PG, Forgert P, DeRoo M, et al (1979) Scintigraphic evaluation of gastrointestinal reflux (GER) in children. J Nucl Med 30:636 (abstract)

46. Piepsz A, Georges B, Perlmutter N (1981) Gastro-oesophageal scintiscanning in children. Pediatr Radiol 11:71-74

47. McVeagh P, Howman-Giles R, Kempt A (1987) Pulmonary aspiration studied by radionuclide milk scanning and barium swallow roentgenography. Am J Dis Child 141:917-921

48. Coben RM, Weintraub A, DiMarino AJ, Cohen S (1994) Gastroesophageal reflux during gastrostomy feeding. Gastroenterology 106:13-18

49. Peracchia A, Bonavina L, Narne S, Segalin A, Antoniazzi L, Marotta G (1988) Minimally invasive surgery for Zenker diverticulum. Analysis of results in 95 consecutive patients. Arch Surg 133:695-700

50. Marotta G, Bonavina L, Voltini F, et al (1997) Radionuclide pharyngo-esophageal transit study before and after transoral Zenker's diverticulum-esophagostomy. Eur J Nucl Med 24:1023

51. Marotta G, Bonavina L, Voltini F, et al (1998) Radionuclide assessment of pharyngo-esophageal emptying before and after transoral Zenker's diverticulum-esophagostomy. J Nucl Med 39:58P

52. Ziessman HA (1996) The gastrointestinal tract. In: Harbert JC, Eckelman WC, Neumann RD (eds) Nuclear medicine. Thieme, New York, pp 585-649

53. Castronovo FP (1986) Gastroesophageal scintiscanning in a pediatric population: dosimetry. J Nucl Med 27:1212-1214

Ambulatory Esophageal pH Monitoring in the Diagnosis of Gastroesophageal Reflux

M. Dinelli[1], D. Fossati[1], and C. Pomari[2]

Introduction

Gastroesophageal reflux disease (GERD) can be defined by any esophageal or extra-esophageal clinical condition or macroscopic or histologic lesion reliably due to measurable GER. Motility disorders of the esophagus and proximal gastrointestinal (GI) tract, increased acid exposure, altered acid perception, and finally, response to drugs inhibiting acid secretion are other relevant aspects of GERD diagnosis [1].

Ambulatory pH monitoring identifies:

- The magnitude of acid exposure and the different patterns of GER (Figs. 1-3),
- The correlation between GER and symptoms, and
- GER response to treatment or the occurrence of drug-induced GER.

Technical Aspects

Electrodes and Recording Units

The electrodes commercially available (Table 1) are sensitive to high concentrations of H^+ and show different physical properties. These electrodes are connected to small-sized recording units which store up to 1 pH measurement per second; data are then processed using appropriate software.

Electrode Placement

The standard placement is 5 cm above the upper margin of the lower esophageal sphincter (LES). This point should be measured by manometry or alterna-

[1]Gastroenterology Unit, Department of Science and Biomedical Technology, San Raffaele University Hospital, Milan, Italy; [2]Lung Department, Bussolengo General Hospital, Bussolengo (Verona), Italy

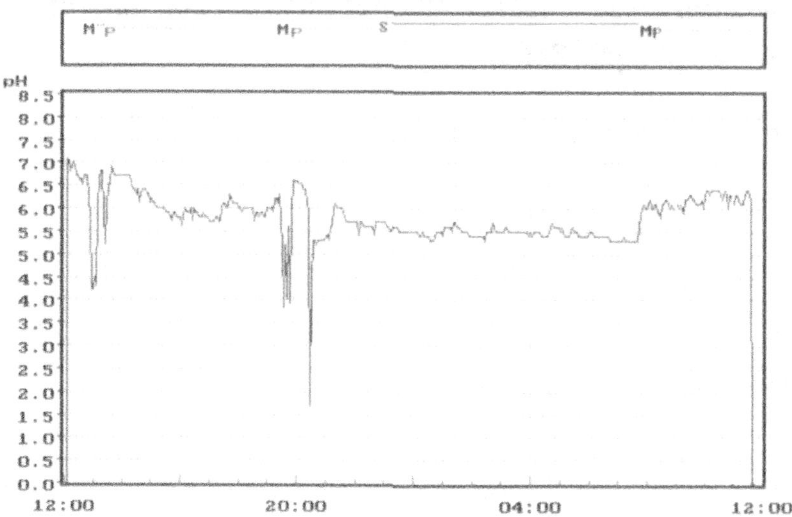

Fig. 1. Esophageal pH profile in a control subject without symptoms and lesions at endoscopy. Rare reflux episodes are present during meals and at postprandial time *(Mp)* while there is no reflux in the nighttime *(S)*. Reflux time is 1.5%

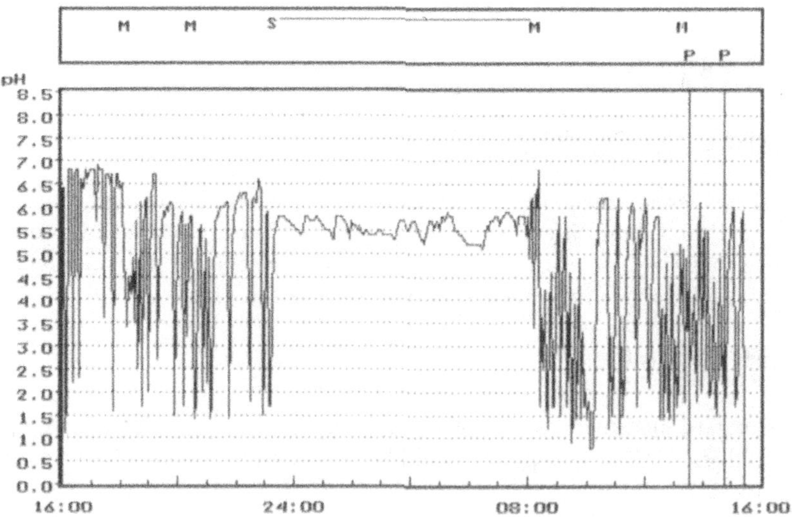

Fig. 2. Esophageal pH profile in a GERD patient with typical upright or daytime reflux not only during the mealtime *(Mp)* but also in the interprandial periods. There is no reflux during the nighttime *(S)*. Two episodes of typical heartburn *(P)* have been recorded. Reflux time is 10% in the 24-hour period, 18% in the daytime and 0% during the night

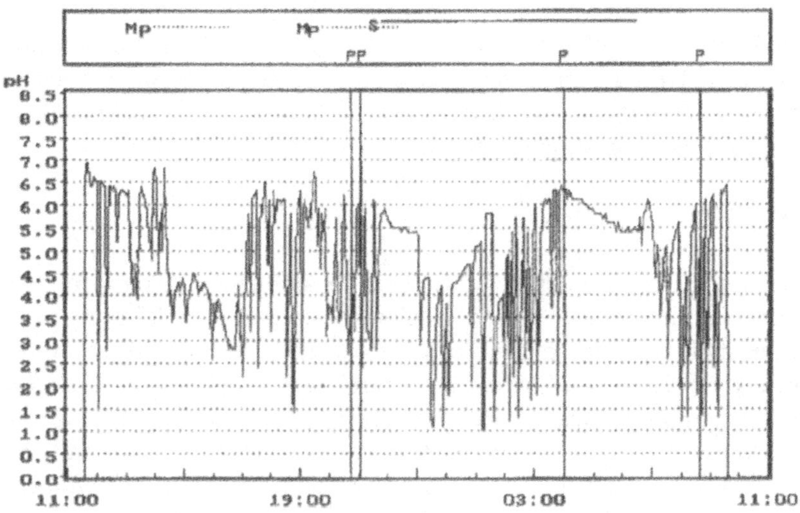

Fig. 3. Esophageal pH profile in a GERD patient with increased reflux both in the daytime (*Mp*, and interprandial) and nighttime (*S*). Typical symptoms (*P*) have been recorded. Reflux time is 25% in the 24-hour period, 21% during the day and 37.4% during the night

Table 1. Properties of standard pH electrodes

	Glass	Antimony
Sensitivity (mV/pH)	50	500
Drift (pH/24 hours)	0.09	0.5
Diameter (mm)	3-4	2
Linearity (pH range)	0-12	0-8
Time of response (s)		
98% of the value	< 25	40
90% of the value	1	20
Lifetime (# recordings)	40	< 10

tively by a LES locator. Other methods such as pull-through or radiological check may not generate sufficiently reliable results [2].

Recording Conditions

There is a large consensus that recording should be free, totally ambulant and lasting 24 h. Drugs interfering with acid secretion or esophago-gastric motility should not be administered if clinical conditions permit.

Data Analysis

Classic DeMeester's pHmetric parameters of analysis [3] are: the percentage of time spent at pH < 4 during the daytime, the nighttime and in the total time of recording, the number of reflux episodes, the number of reflux episode lasting > 5 min, and the longest reflux episode.

Reflux Episodes

The pHmetric definition of "reflux episode" is ambiguous. A reflux episode can be defined as an abrupt drop of pH below the cutoff of pH 4, lasting at least 20 s. pH threshold was chosen arbitrarily but the distribution of pH measurements in healthy controls shows that the pH rarely drops below this cutoff (Fig. 4). Moreover, symptoms occurrence and severity of mucosal damage are strictly related to pH. The duration of pH drops can be indeed shorter, and episodes lasting less than 20 s but low enough in pH, may contribute to abnormal acid exposure. Finally, the number of reflux episodes should not be considered reliable or diagnostic because of potential artifacts due to sample frequency [4, 5].

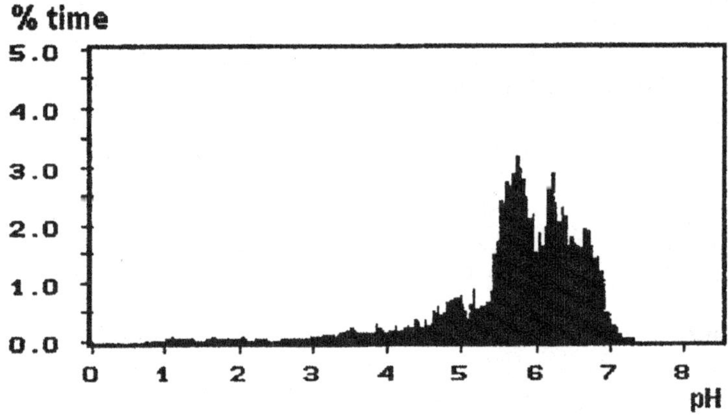

Fig. 4. Frequency distribution of pH data at different pH levels in a control-subjects population (personal data). Note that pH rarely drops below pH 4

Acid Exposure

The contact time or reflux time (RT), expressed in minutes below pH 4, and percentage RT are considered the most sensitive and reliable quantitative measures of GER [2, 4, 5]. RT can be calculated for different periods of interest (meals, night, day). The purpose of RT is identify subjects with abnormal acid exposure. However, problems arise in:

- Defining a cutoff or the upper limit of normality, as shown by the great variability of literature data (Table 2) [6-10] and by the confusion in statistical approach (pH data are not normally distributed so that an appropriate description requires non-parametric descriptors);
- Evaluating the predictive value of the test in clinical practice; GERD definition is wide and covers esophageal and extra-esophageal symptoms and lesions. Patients may have normal acid exposure but be abnormally sensitive to acid, or they may have macroscopic esophagitis but normal RT. From a Bayesian point of view, the definition of upper limit for acid exposure is greatly influenced by the population in which the test is applied. Sensitivity and specificity are quite good comparing controls and subjects with esophagitis, but are disappointingly low in the endoscopy-negative GERD patients.

Table 2. Reference values for acid exposure (RT) and sensitivity/specificity figures for GERD patients with and without esophagitis. Note the variability of upper limit of normality, the different statistical approaches and the different performances of the tests in patients with symptoms and mucosal damage and in patients with symptoms but no esophagitis. (Modified from [2])

	Controls (n)	Statistical approach	RT (% at pH < 4)	GERD patients	
				With esophagitis Se/Sp (%)	Without esophagitis Se/Sp (%)
Vitale et al. [6]	22	Mean ± 3 SD	7.2	77/91	64/91
Schindlebeck et al. [7]	42	ROCs	7	89/93	NA
Johnsson et al. [8]	20	95th percentile	3.4	87/97	NA
Mattioli et al. [9]	20	Mean ± 2 SD	5	92/100	0/100
Dinelli et al. [10]	20	ROCs	5	80/81	63/81

SD, standard deviations; *ROCs*, receving operator characteristics; *Se/Sp*, sensitivity/specificity; *NA*, data not available

Reflux Area or "Area Under pH 4"

In the definition of reflux episode, the pH drop is one of the two dimensions causing problems. Much attention has been focused on the duration (or contact time) of reflux episodes. Attempts to include pH in the calculation of acid exposure have been sporadically reported in the literature [11, 12]. The basic concept is, however, that the integral of the curve representing pH below pH 4 can measure this bidimensional nature of GER. We have studied this nonconventional quantitative evaluation of GER [10] searching for optimal cutoffs for RT and area under pH 4 (AU4) curve (Table 3, Fig. 5). We compared 20 healthy subjects with no symptoms or lesions and 42 GERD patients, 18 of which had esophagitis and 24 had typical symptoms (heartburn). The cutoffs obtained by receiving operator characteristic (ROC) analysis were prospectively tested in a sample of 110 patients with GERD (55 with esophagitis). AU4, which identified all the patients with abnormal RT and also 32% of patients with RT within normal limits, had the best predictive value (Table 4). Using this approach, asthma researchers [13] found that AU4 was able to identify methacholine-positive subjects with GER but normal RT. AU4 also seemed to be correlated to the methacholine response (Table 5). An example of a typical AU4-positive patient is shown in Fig. 6.

Table 3. Personal data on reference values for RT and AU4. Values are expressed as median (range). Cutoffs derived by ROC analysis have been compared and AU4 gave the best performance in discriminating controls and GERD patients

	Controls (n = 20)	GERD, no esophagitis (n = 24)	GERD esophagitis (n = 18)	ROC analysis		
				Cutoff	Area	SE
RT	1.9 (0.1-6)	4.4 (1.3-34.8)	10.5 (2.6-58.8)	5.1	0.899	0.038
AU4	13.3 (0.5-55.6)	72.8 (7.6-726)	134.7 (42.2-1445)	36.1	0.935*	0.03

*$p = 0.038$

Table 4. Cutoffs for RT and AU4 (personal data, see Table 3) tested in a sample of 110 GERD patients (55 with esophagitis) submitted to esophageal pH monitoring. AU4 identified all patients with abnormal RT (> 5.1%) and 10 of 31 (32%) patients with normal RT (< 5.1%)

	RT	AU4
Sensitivity	71.8	80.9*
Specificity	81.2	81.2
Predictive positive value	96.3	96.7
Predictive negative value	29.5	38.2

*$\chi^2 = 8.1$ ($p < 0.005$)

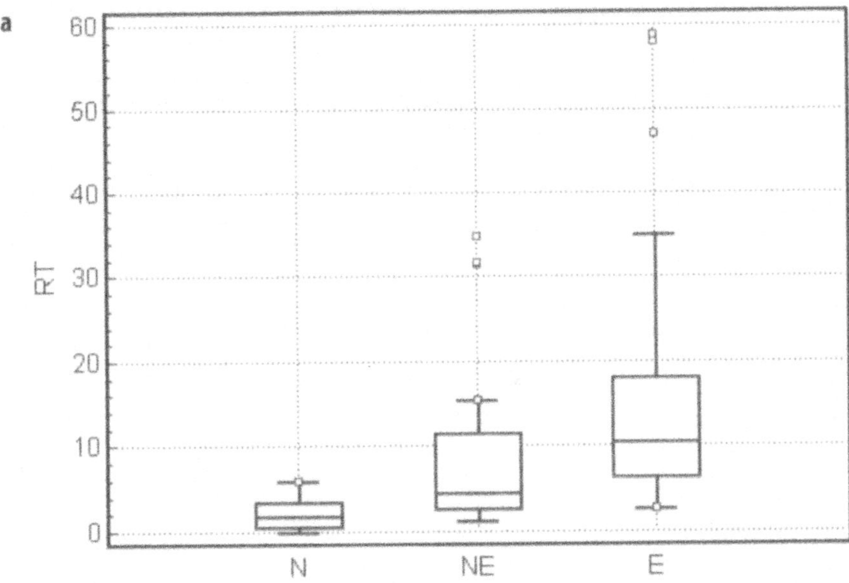

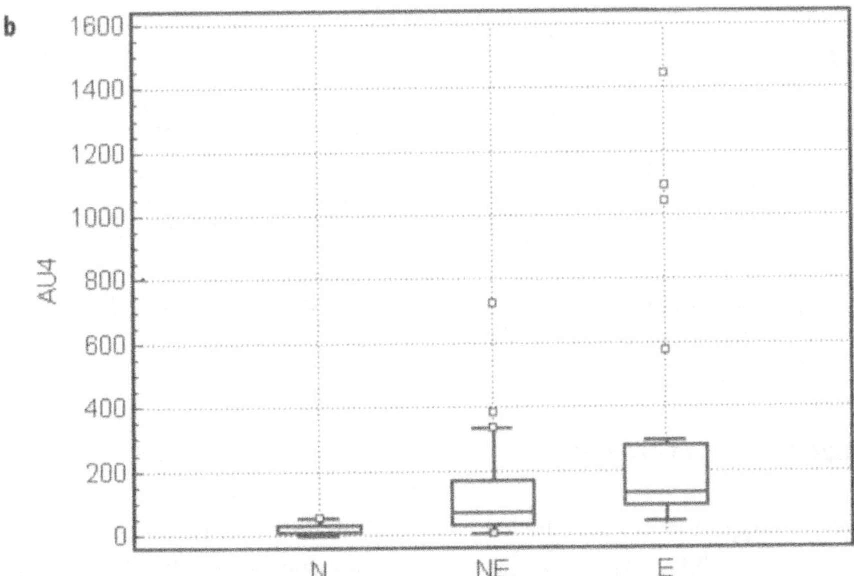

Fig. 5a,b. *Box and Whisker graph.* Median, 25th and 75th percentiles, and exceeding values of pH data in control subjects (*N*), GERD patients without esophagitis (*NE*) and GERD patients with erosive esophagitis (*E*) are shown. **a** Reflux time (*RT*). **b** Area under pH 4 (*AU4*)

Table 5. Response to methacholine (MCh) in patients with persistent cough suspected to be GER-related, divided according to pH monitoring results. Significant response to MCh was assessed only in patients with abnormal acid exposure measured by RT or AU4 ($p < 0.001$ versus patients with normal RT and normal AU4). AU4 selects patients with abnormal MCh response even if RT is within normal limits. (Modified from [9])

	Normal RT and AU4 (n = 9)	Normal RT and increased AU4 (n = 9)	Increased RT and AU4 (n = 9)
PD_{20} of FEV_1	1167 ± 272.3	208.8 ± 76.3	133.5 ± 37.2

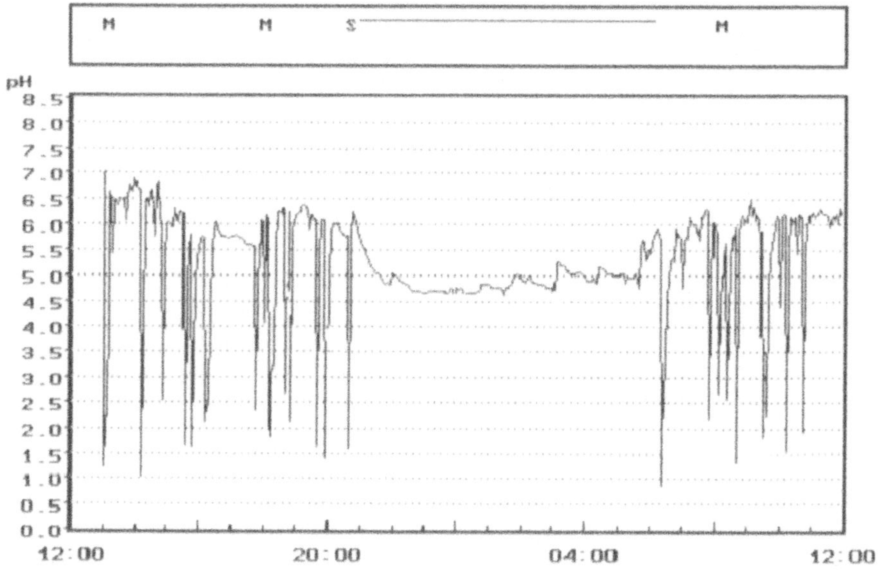

Fig. 6. Typical esophageal pH profile in a patient with erosive esophagitis and 24-hour RT within the normal range (3.1%) but abnormal AU4 (57.7 pH x min)

Symptom-Reflux Correlation

A relevant aspect of pH monitoring is the potential demonstration of a correlation between reflux episodes and symptoms reported by patients. A one-to-one correlation, however, does not exist and different temporal windows for a "significant" correlation have been published. Statistical manipulations or indexes suggested are:
- *Symptom index* [14], obtained by dividing the reflux-related symptoms by the total number of symptoms reported. This approach does not consider

the total number of reflux episodes and may cause false-positive diagnoses. To circumvent this problem, the *symptom sensitivity index* [15] was developed; this is defined as the percentage of symptom-associated reflux episodes. In both indexes the cutoff for positive score is arbitrary.

- *Symptom-association probability index* [16] that compares in a contingency table 2-minute periods with symptoms and no refluxes, refluxes but no symptoms, symptoms and refluxes, and no symptoms nor refluxes. This index measures the mere casual association between symptoms and pH drops.

These statistical approaches do not include, however, the evaluation of pain perception behaviour. Moreover, some researchers described the possibility that prolonged acidification makes the esophagus sensitive to relatively small quantities of acid or to pH drops not necessary below pH 4. This could explain the occurrence of symptoms (the concept of acid load or burden) [17].

Dual-Channel pH Monitoring

To test the hypothesis of proximal reflux in respiratory conditions suspected to be GER-related (ear, nose and throat - ENT - or pulmonary disorders), dual-channel recording with proximal electrode close to or above the upper esophageal sphincter has become popular in the past years (Fig. 7). This approach seems to be attractive but until now no standard technique no analysis consensus has been developed either in ENT or in asthma studies [2].

Recently, an Italian multicentre study [18] was conducted in 22 healthy controls, in 114 patients with typical GER symptoms, and in 116 patients with ENT complaints all submitted to dual-channel pH monitoring with the proximal electrode 1-3 cm below the upper esophageal sphincter, determined manometrically. Data analysis (Table 6) revealed that:

Table 6. GISMAD Italian study on proximal reflux

		Controls (n = 22)	GERD patients (n = 114)	ENT patients (n = 116)
Proximal RT		$0.1 \pm 0.1^*$	1.3 ± 2.2	1.3 ± 2.2
Ratio (%) proximal/distal reflux episodes	24-hour	16.1 ± 20.4	20.9 ± 24.2	$28.6 \pm 35.6^{**}$
	Night	1.9 ± 6.7	14.6 ± 22.7	$37.5 \pm 89.4^{**}$
Proximal RT according to distal RT	Distal normal	–	0.2 ± 0.2	0.4 ± 0.6
	Distal abnormal	–	$1.8 \pm 2.6^*$	$2.4 \pm 3.3^*$

$^*p < 0.01$; $^{**}p < 0.05$

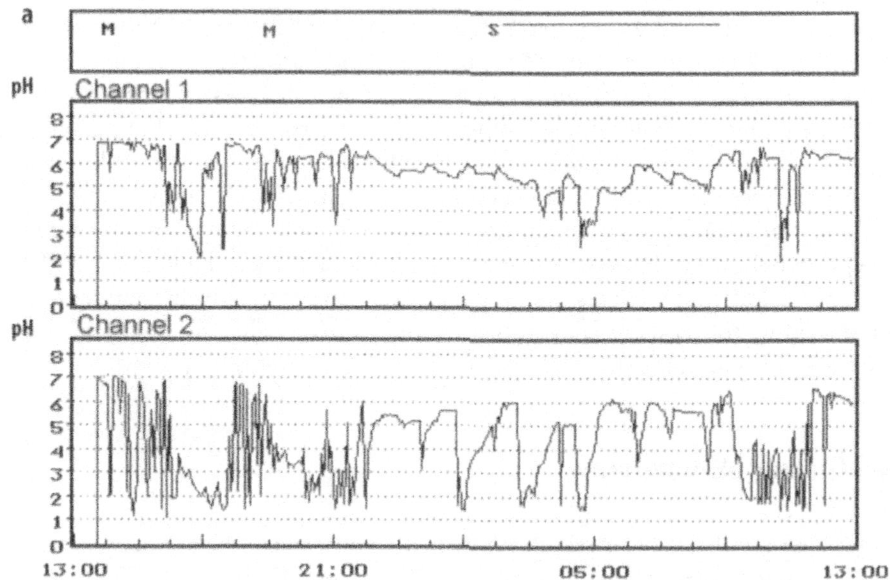
a
M   M   S
pH   Channel 1
8
7
6
5
4
3
2
1
0
pH   Channel 2
8
7
6
5
4
3
2
1
0
13:00   21:00   05:00   13:00

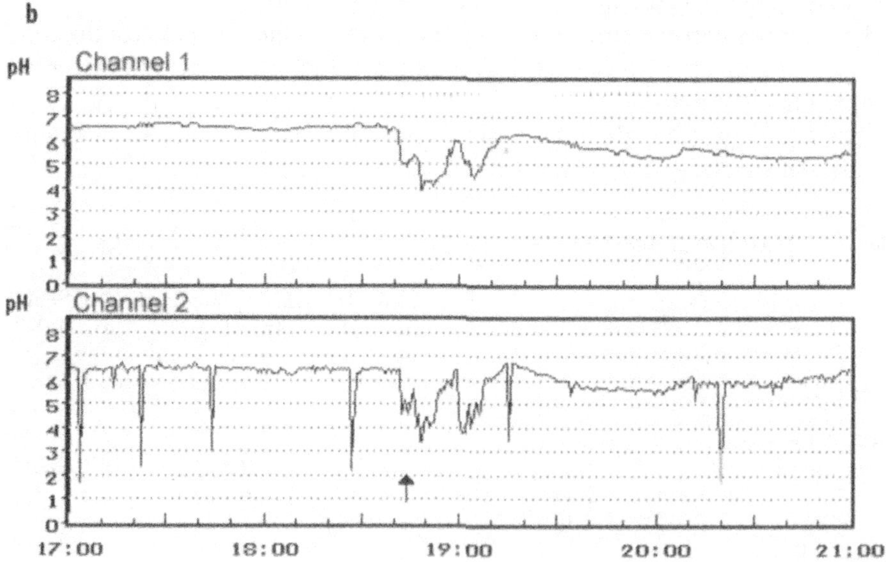
b
pH   Channel 1
8
7
6
5
4
3
2
1
0
pH   Channel 2
8
7
6
5
4
3
2
1
0
17:00   18:00   19:00   20:00   21:00

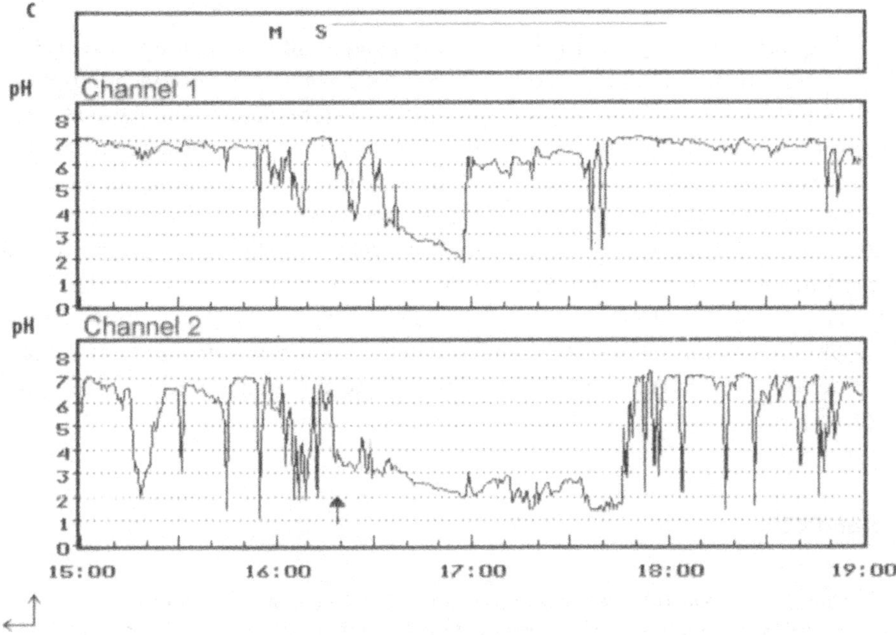

Fig. 7a-c. *Dual-channel esophageal pH recording.* Channel 1 was connected to proximal electrode, 1-3 cm below the upper esophageal sphincter and channel 2 to distal electrode in standard position. **a** Patient with erosive esophagitis and no respiratory complaints. Proximal extension of acid reflux is a common event but patient does not feel it. **b** Patient with chronic cough and normal esophageal mucosa at endoscopy, where distal acid exposure is not revelant but proximal extension correlates to symptoms (*arrow*). **c** Patient with asthma and erosive esophagitis where both distal and promimal acid exposures are prominent, and wheezing (*arrow*) is related to prolonged to supine postprandial reflux episodes with impaired clearance at both distal and proximal sites of recording

- Proximal GER is rare in healthy controls but a common phenomenon in both typical GERD and ENT patients.
- The entity of proximal GER, measured by the ratio of proximal/distal reflux episodes, is greater in ENT patients, if compared with typical GERD patients. These latter patients, not surprisingly, have a greater distal GER than both ENT patients and controls.
- Proximal GER seems to be unrelated to the presence or severity of esophagitis or laryngitis.

Conclusions

Esophageal pH monitoring is a sensitive test for detecting acid GER. Appropriate technical equipment and recording standards should be applied. The predictive value of the test is greatly influenced by the clinical context. Acid exposure, classically measured by reflux time, is a simple, sensitive and reliable quantitative parameter of analysis, but the area under pH 4 (AU4) seems to be the best discriminating tool in this field. Symptom analysis is far from standardized and problems regarding temporal correlation, statistical evaluation of symptoms-reflux association, and pathophysiological basis of symptoms perception are not solved. Dual-channel pH monitoring has become popular in the field of GER-linked respiratory complaints but further interdisciplinary research is advisable to clarify the pathophysiology and the interpretation of the tests applied.

References

1. Dent J (1998) Gastro-oesophageal reflux disease. Digestion 59:433-445
2. Karhilas PJ, Quigley EMM (1996) Clinical esophageal pH recording: a technical review for practice guideline development. Gastroenterology 110:1982-1996
3. Johnson LF, DeMeester TR (1974) 24-hour pH monitoring of the distal esophagus. A quantitative measure of gastroesophageal reflux disease. Am J Gastroenterol 62:325-332
4. DeCaestecker JS, Heading RC (1990) Esophageal pH monitoring. Gastroenterol Clin North Am 19:645-669
5. Galmiche JP, Scarpignato C (1994) Esophageal pH monitoring In: Scarpignato C, Galmiche JP (eds) Functional evaluation in esophageal disease (Frontiers in gastrointestinal research, vol. 22). Karger, Basel, pp 71-108
6. Vitale GC, Cheadle WG, Sadek S, et al (1984) Computerized 24-hour ambulatory esophageal pH monitoring and esophagogastroduodenoscopy in the reflux patient. Ann Surg 20:724-728
7. Schindlebeck NE, Heinrich C, Konig A, et al (1987) Optimal thresholds, sensitivity and specificity of long-term pH-metry for the detection of gastroesophageal reflux disease. Gastroenterology 93:85-90
8. Johnsson F, Joelsson B, Isberg PE (1987) Ambulatory 24-hour intraesophageal pH monitoring in the diagnosis of gastroesophageal reflux disease. Gut 28:1145-1150
9. Mattioli S, Pilotti V, Spangaro M, et al (1989) Reliability of 24-hour home esophageal pH-monitoring in diagnosis of gastroesophageal reflux. Dig Dis Sci 34:71-78
10. Dinelli M, Passaretti S, DiFrancia I, et al (1999) Area under pH 4: a more sensitive parameter for the quantitative analysis of esophageal acid exposure in adults. Am J Gastroenterol (submitted)
11. Vandenplas Y, Francx-Goossens A, Pipeleers-Marichal M, et al (1989) Area under pH 4: advantage of a new parameter in the interpretation of esophageal pH monitoring data in infants. J Pediatr Gastroenterol Nutr 9:934-939
12. Tovar JA, Izquierdo MA, Eizaguirre I (1991) The area under pH curve: a single figure parameter representative of esophageal acid exposure. J Pediatr Surg 26:163-167
13. Pomari C, Dinelli M, Passaretti S, Micheletto C, Dal Negro R (1997) Bronchial

hyperreactivity and gastroesophageal reflux (GER): a more sensitive parameter for detecting the extent of acid exposure. Chest 112:114 (abstract)

14. Wiener GJ, Richter JE, Copper JB, et al (1988) The symptom index: a clinically important parameter of ambulatory 24-hour esophageal pH monitoring. Am J Gastroenterol 38:358-361

15. Breumelhof R, Smout AJPM (1991) The symptom sensitivtiy index: a valuable additional parameter in 24-hour esophageal pH recording. Am J Gastroenterol 86:160-164

16. Weusten BLAM, Roelofs JMM, Akkermanns LMA, et al (1994) The symptom-association probability: an improved method for symptom analysis of 24-hour esophageal pH data. Gastroenterology 107:1741-1745

17. Janssen J, Vantrappen G, Vos R, Ghillebert G (1992) The acid burden over an extended period preceeding a reflux episode is a major determinant in the development of heartburn. Gastroenterology 102:A90

18. Baldi F, Brancaccio ML, Cappiello R, et al (1997) Proximal G-E reflux in patients with unexplained otolaryngologic (ORL) symptoms. A multicenter study in Italy, AGA 1997. DOW Abstract Book, A-117

Diagnostic Techniques
for Assessing Pulmonary Involvement

Lung Function and Bronchial Hyperreactivity

R.W. Dal Negro and C. Pomari

Introduction

Gastroesophageal reflux (GER) is a digestive dysfunction which frequently occurs in healthy people to some extent, and is then regarded as a physiological event in these cases. GER occurrence frequently combines with the onset of one or more respiratory symptoms of different severities, creating a situation which may assume a significant clinical impact [1]. In these cases, cough and wheezing are the most important clinical signs, and those most frequently and spontaneously referred to GER occurrence by the patient. Unfortunately, except in a few paradigmatic circumstances, the cause-effect relationship between the occurrences of GER and of respiratory symptoms is still difficult to assess in the majority of cases, and can only be presumed or established on the basis of the patient's clinical history in many cases.

Up to now, conventional pulmonary function tests did not prove sensitive and specific enough in characterizing GER-related respiratory troubles; particularly, spirometrical parameters which are routinary used for detecting airway patency did not provide their usual diagnostic support. At present, the conventional assessment of nonspecific bronchial hyperresponsiveness also does not consent a clear identification of specific and reliable GER-related functional patterns of response.

Data from the literature frequently lead to conflicting results, likely due to the lack of precise clinico-functional models. In 1981 [2], a 10% increase in total respiratory resistance was assessed after esophageal acid infusion in asthmatic subjects previously characterized by a Bernstein positive test. A different study carried out during the same year in asthmatic subjects with GER proved that esophageal acidification causes only a 0.2 l decrease in vital capacity and a 0.9% increase in alveolar plateau [3]. Another study investigated the effect of esophageal acid infusion in 15 nocturnal asthmatics by measuring respiratory flow, tidal volume, and airflow resistance during sleep [4]: no significant acute or sustained changes in airflow resistance were found when acid was present in the esophagus.

Lung Department, Bussolengo General Hospital, Bussolengo (Verona), Italy

Because previous studies failed to check for microaspiration, studies were performed using state-of-the-art pulmonary techniques and dual-electrode esophageal pH testing (Fig. 1) [5, 6]. Peak expiratory flow rate (PEFR) was found to decrease during acid infusion into the esophagus of normal control subjects, asthmatics with GER, asthmatics without GER, and subjects with GER alone [5]. Esophageal acid clearance improved PEFR in all groups except in the asthma-with-GER group, which had a further decrease in PEFR. These effects proved independent of the Bernstein test result or of proximal esophageal acid exposure, which is considered a prerequisite for confirming the occurrence of microaspiration [5]. Moreover, subjects in the asthma-with-GER group showed also a substantial increase in specific airway resistance during esophageal acid infusion, which continued to increase despite the intervention of an efficient acid clearance mechanism [5]. Furthermore, while decreasing PEFR, a significant increase in airway resistance was also observed in subjects belonging to the asthma-with-GER group when lying in supine position: once again it was unaffected by spontaneous acid clearance [7]. Vagolytic doses of i.v. atropine partially ablated this response, suggesting the relevant contribution of a vago-mediated mechanism (i.e. reflex) in determining these functional phenomena [6].

More recently, simultaneous tracheal and esophageal pH monitoring was performed in four patients with severe asthma [8]. Thirty-seven episodes of esophageal reflux lasting more than 5 min were observed, and five of these episodes were associated with a remarkable fall in tracheal pH. PEFR decreased

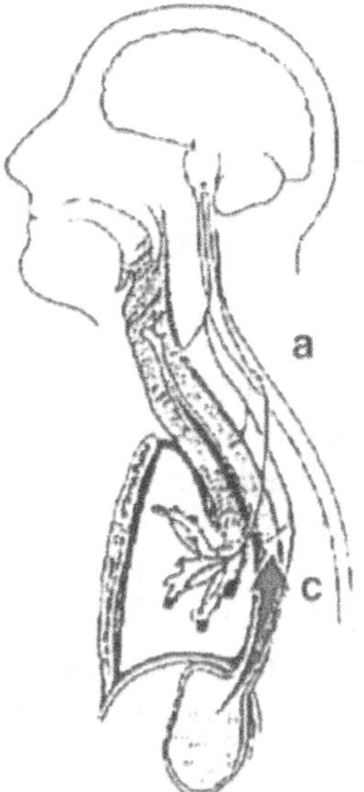
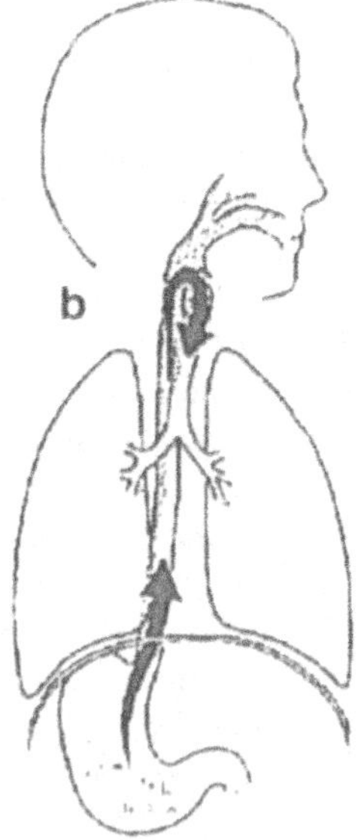

Fig. 1. Three are the potential mechanisms which can induce or impair respiratory troubles in asthmatic subjects with GER, and schematically: (**a**) the occurrence of a vagally mediated reflex; (**b**) the microaspiration of acid gastric content; (**c**) the GER-induced heightening of bronchial hyperreactivity

by 84 l/min when both esophageal and tracheal acidification were assessed, and by 8 l/min when only esophageal acidification was confirmed [8].

In order to reliably interpret data, which can sometimes appear conflicting indeed, it should be remembered that in asthma patients with GER esophageal acid stimulation can impair respiratory symptoms not only via the directly induced bronchial obstruction, but also by exalting the level of nonspecific airway hyperresponsiveness (such as methacholine, histamine, and isocapnic hyperventilation) [9, 10].

The effect of esophageal acid infusion on expiratory flow was investigated in asthmatics with and without GER who were challenged with voluntary isocapnic hyperventilation of dry air and methacholine (MCh) [10]. Perfusion of acid (i.e. HCl) into the distal esophagus caused slight but significant bronchoconstriction in asthmatic subjects with GER, and enhanced the bronchoconstriction produced by isocapnic hyperventilation and MCh in asthmatics, independently of the presence of GER [10]. The authors suggested that the stimulation of esophageal acid-sensitive receptors could affect the cholinergic bronchial tone. The firing of a vago-mediated reflex was then presumed, and the hypothesis that GER can aggravate asthma by enhancing the nonspecific bronchial hyperresponsiveness was further emphasized [10]. Previous evidence for the occurrence of an acid-induced, vago-mediated esophago-bronchial reflex [11] had been assessed a few years earlier when atropine pre-treatment was found to minimize the significant reduction in airflow and arterial oxygen saturation in 136 subjects caused by esophageal acid infusion [2].

Further to the effects of GER-induced acid microaspiration and of vago-mediated reflexes on lung function, changes in lung mechanics were also presumed to affect the function of the gastroesophageal tract. The exalted negativity of pleural pressure due to the occurrence of spontaneous airway obstruction during asthma may substantially increase the thoraco-abdominal pressure gradient, and thereby promote the occurrence of reflux episodes [12]. In addition, the overinflation and the air trapping phenomena operating in these circumstances might lead to flattening of the diaphragm, up to the potential (and sometimes remarkable) impairment of its antireflux barrier effect.

The MCh-induced airflow limitation was also investigated from this point of view. In a study carried out more than ten years ago on asthma patients with GER, MCh-induced airway narrowing coexisted with longer lasting periods of reflux as compared with the baseline condition [13]. On the contrary, a much more controlled investigation carried out a few years ago on mild asthmatics with GER and differently graded in terms of bronchial response to MCh (PD_{20} FEV1[1] ranging < 100-1600 µg), documented that the MCh-induced bronchoconstriction did not cause any significant impairment of GER at all, both in terms of number and severity of reflux episodes [14]. Moreover, a remarkable, even though not statistically significant, reduction in GER episodes was documented in the same

---

[1] PD_{20} FEV1 = the provocative dose (µg) of bronchial challenge which is able to induce a 20% decrease from baseline of forced expiratory volume in 1 s

study after MCh challenge: this effect was related to the direct cholinergic effect of MCh on the lower esophageal sphincter (LES) tone (Table 1) [14].

As previously mentioned, spirometrical indices have not yet revealed a functional bronchial response which can be regarded as peculiar for GER-related respiratory dysfunction. On the other hand, commonly used nonspecific bronchial challenges (such as MCh, histamine, or physical stimuli) directly or indirectly stimulate different structural targets along airways (e.g. smooth muscles, epithelial and mucosal tissues, neural endings and receptors, bronchial vasculature), and several functional indicators (not only those related to the airway flow limitation, and mainly dependent on muscular function) may be influenced. These indicators are preferentially used to more completely investigate the effects of these challenges [15, 16].

A few years ago, the noninvasive transcutaneous monitoring of respiratory PO_2 and PCO_2 proved sensitive in assessing the early airway response to nonspecific bronchial challenges such as ultrasonic nebulized distilled water (UNDW), also

Table 1. Different degrees of MCh-induced acute bronchoconstriction did not cause any significant impairment of GER (neither in terms of number nor of severity of GER episodes) when the bronchial challenge was performed during gastroesophageal pH monitoring. (Modified from [14])

	Mean pH		GER episodes		Duration pH < 4	
	Before	After	Before	After	Before	After
Nonresponders	5.3 ± 0.7	5.4 ± 0.4	2.2 ± 1.6	1.3 ± 0.7	133.3 ± 82.7	80.0 ± 48.1
Mild responders (Mean PD_{20} FEV1 = 490 µg $\pm$ 5.3)	6.4 ± 0.1	6.3 ± 0.1	0.3 ± 0.2	0.2 ± 0.1	20.0 ± 16.3	13.3 ± 13.0
Heavy responders (Mean PD_{20} FEV1 = 81.8 µg $\pm$ 14.9)	5.8 ± 0.4	5.8 ± 0.3	0.5 ± 0.2	0.3 ± 0.2	36.6 ± 22.3	17.3 ± 11.3

t paired tests before and after MCh for all variables always not significant

when spirometry was unresponsive [16]. In contrast to normal controls, atopic asthmatics showed a peculiar biphasic time-course of PO_2 and PCO_2 during and following UNDW inhalation by means of this functional model. The first phase was characterized by a sudden, although transient (3-4 min duration), hypocapnic response; the second showed a delayed, but remarkable and long-lasting hypoxemic response, with a 6-7 min duration following the end of inhalation of the hypo-osmolar challenge (Fig. 2). The respiratory events which correspond to this particular time-course of functional indices were: a significant hyperventilation (likely due to the stimulation of mucosal triggers) in the first phase, which precedes the occurrence of a substantial V_A/Q_c mismatch in

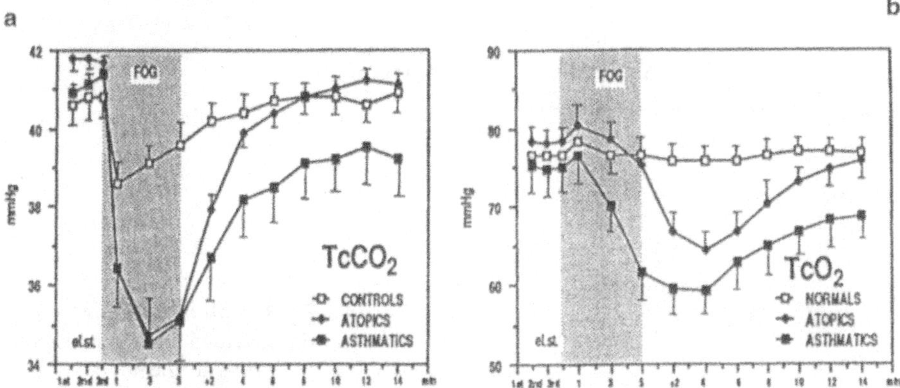

Fig. 2a,b. Noninvasive time-course of **a** TcCO$_2$ (transcutaneous CO$_2$ partial pressure in mm Hg), and of **b** TcO$_2$ (transcutaneous O$_2$ partial pressure in mm Hg) during and following fog challenge (hypoosmolar bronchial challenge with ultrasonic nebulized distilled water, UNDW) in normal subjects, in atopic asthmatics, and in subjects with atopic rhinitis (mean ± SE). Despite normal controls, a sudden hypocapnic response systematically precedes a longer lasting hypoxemic phase in atopic subjects, even though to a lesser extent in atopic rhinitis. (Modified from [16, 18])

the second phase of the response. Even though to a lesser extent, this particular pattern of functional changes was also assessed in atopic rhinitics who never experienced wheezing episodes and proved absolutely unresponsive in spirometrical terms to UNDW inhalation [18]. This functional behavior of respiratory gases, specific indeed, lead us to propose the existence of a transitional phase between normality and the asthmatic range of bronchial reactivity, which could discriminate susceptible individuals who would be otherwise neglected treatment.

Because of the higher sensitivity and reproducibility of this method, the hyperreactive response pattern of GER subjects to UNDW was investigated in different clinical situations, such as in mild asthma and GER, and in persistent cough and GER [17, 19]. In contrast to atopic asthmatics [16], in these circumstances the hyperreactive pattern of response was characterized only by a dramatic and long-lasting hypocapnic phase (such as hyperventilation) following UNDW inhalation, without any hypoxemic effect (Fig. 3) [17]. This functional event proved peculiar only in the presence of GER, as the calculated specificity was higher than 82% when GER- and non-GER subjects were compared from this point of view [20]. Even though to a lesser extent, this particular response to UNDW was also confirmed in asymptomatic GER subjects without any previous respiratory complaint (Fig. 4) [21].

These results contributed to further emphasize the crucial role of acid GER in modulating the hyperreactive airway response to physical stimuli (such as to hypo-osmolar challenge), the exhalted triggering of airway reflexes (via C fibers) being the pathogenetic mechanism suggested in these cases [22].

The primary role of GER was further highlighted by experimental physiological studies carried out to investigate the activities of acid-sensitive receptors (see also chapter by Geppetti et al., in the present volume). When these

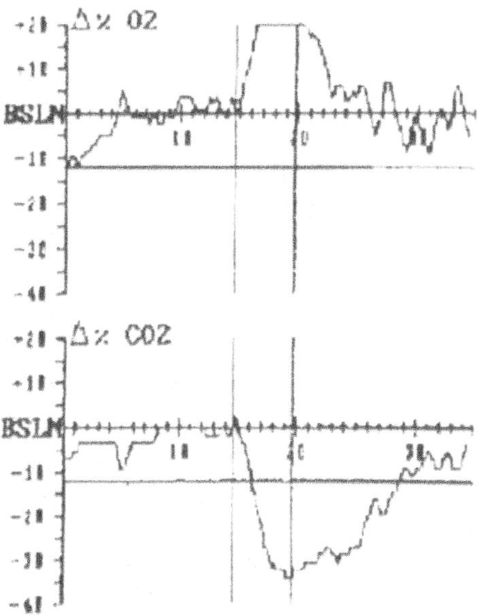

Fig. 3. Asthmatic subjects with documented acid GER respond with only a marked and long-lasting hyperventilation (such as transcutaneous hypocapnia) to UNDW. Despite atopics, this pattern of response (characterized by only negligible hypoxemic effects) is peculiar in these cases, with high specificity (see text). A paradigmatic example

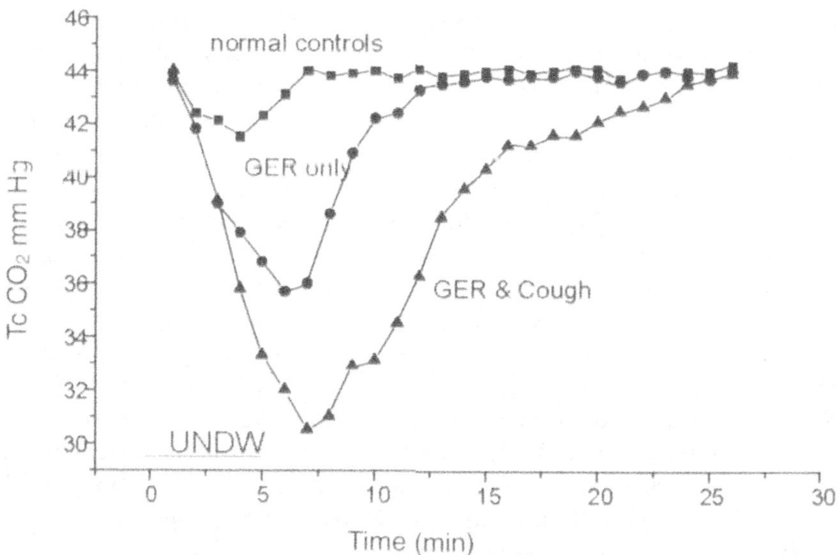

Fig. 4. Noninvasive time-courses of $TcCO_2$ (transcutaneous CO_2 partial pressure in mm Hg) assessed in response to UNDW in normal controls, in subjects with documented acid GER without any respiratory complaint and in nonatopic GER subjects with persistent cough. Despite normals, the longlasting hypocapnic response proves the peculiar functional indicator of GER presence; when respiratory signs (such as cough) are combined with GER this specific pattern of bronchial response is much more pronounced

esophageal receptors are sensitized by adequate stimuli, conventional challenges and indicators provide useful diagnostic support, even in clinical models. In fact, in subjects originally unresponsive to MCh and characterized by persistent cough and acid GER, the previous (15 min) ingestion of an acid drink (120 ml; pH 3.5-3.7) caused a significant increase in the spirometrical response to MCh (PD$_{20}$ FEV1 from 2578.0 µg (SE 401.4) to 407.9 µg (SE 79.3); $p < 0.002$), the acid drink working as a specific esophageal challenge in these cases [19]. These pathophysiological events were affected to some extent by drugs currently used to control GER. These drugs actively modify the esophageal acid condition existing in these subjects.

In a controlled study vs. placebo, the long-term administration of only a prokinetic drug (cisapride 30 mg tid for 30 days) was able to significantly modify the hyperreactive response to UNDW in patients with persistent cough and GER: when compared with pretreatment conditions, the marked UNDW-induced hyperventilation was substantially reduced in all subjects, while cough was minimized [23] only following the active treatment (trend analysis between curves and shapes, $p < 0.001$). The effectiveness of cisapride, a drug affecting only esophageal contractility without any documented effect in modifying the esophageal acid environment, was then presumed to be related to the enhancement of the esophageal clearance efficacy in these circumstances, so leading to the substantial reduction of the esophageal acid contact time, which is in fact greatly increased in the majority of GER patients [1].

The respiratory effects of the pharmacological-induced gastroesophageal acid control were also investigated vs. placebo in cross-over, double-blind studies with proton pump inhibitors. In contrast to placebo, an 8-week treatment with omeprazole (20 mg o.d.) systematically reduced the bronchial hyper-responsiveness to MCh in mild, nonatopic asthmatics with GER (PD$_{20}$ FEV1 from 460.1 µg (SE 104.0) to 1201.9 µg (SE 247.8); $p < 0.02$) [24]. On the other hand, in a previous controlled double-blind, cross-over vs. placebo study, a 4-week daily treatment with the same therapeutic regimen was indicated as highly effective in systematically improving the original airway obstruction in moderate-to-severe asthmatics with GER (mean FEV1 from 59.3% (SE 3.2) to 71.6% (SE 4.2); $p < 0.03$) [25]. The same therapeutic regimen was also confirmed to be effective in improving PEFR in documented asthma and GER [26].

The crucial role of the GER-induced esophageal acidification in causing asthma-like respiratory effects (both in terms of pathophysiologic and clinical outcomes) was further confirmed when considering the beneficial effects obtained with the newer molecules belonging to this class of drugs, particularly with pantoprazole.

In a recent controlled study vs. placebo, a selected sample of very mild, non-atopic asthmatics originally unresponsive to MCh showed a heightened bronchial hyperresponse when esophageal stimulation with a standardized acid drink preceded (by 15 min) the MCh challenge [27]. Despite placebo, a 3-day short course of pantoprazole (40 mg o.d.) restored the original MCh unresponsiveness in all subjects [27].

Table 2. In contrast to normals, nonatopic asthmatics+GER and nonatopic subjects with persistent cough+GER show a substantial increase in eosinophilic inflammation, even though to a lesser extent in the latter subset of patients

	FEV$_1$ (% predicted)	PD$_{20}$ FEV$_1$ (µg)	IS-ECP (µg/l)	s-ECP (µg/l)	EOS (% total leucocytes)
Nonatopic asthma +GER (n = 8)	90.7 ± 3.0	180.0 ± 162	1713.7 ± 845.8*	18.9 ± 7.8*	8.6 ± 2.5*
Persistent cough +GER (n = 8)	93.2 ± 3.3	> 3150	203.2 ± 37.9*	8.3 ± 0.8*	4.0 ± 0.8*
Normal volunteers (n = 8)	89.9 ± 7.3	2889 ± 226	33.3 ± 11.2	4.1 ± 1.9	2.7 ± 1.1

IS-ECP, level of eosinophilic cationic protein in induced sputum; *s-ECP,* serum level of eosinophilic cationic protein; *EOS,* eosinophil count in blood
* *t* test *p* < 0.05

Recently, remarkable increases in eosinophil cell count and eosinophilic cationic protein (ECP) were also assessed in spontaneous or induced sputum from nonatopic GER subjects [28, 29]. The extent of eosinophilic bronchial inflammation proved related to the extent of MCh hyperresponsiveness and to the clinical severity of respiratory signs in these cases (Table 2) [29], as the ECP level and eosinophil count in bronchial secretions from nonatopic asthmatics with GER were similar to those found in atopic asthmatics of the same severity [30].

When confirmed, these recent results will further support the strict relation ship between pathological esophageal acidification and the occurrence (or per-sistency) of GER-induced respiratory changes of inflammatory origin.

References

1. Irwin RS, Zawacki JK, Curley FJ, et al (1989) Chronic cough as the sole presenting manifestation of gastroesophageal reflux. Am Rev Respir Dis 140:1294-1300
2. Mansfield LE, Hameister HH, Spaulding MS, et al (1981) The role of the vagus nerve in airway narrowing caused by intraesophageal hydrocloric acid provocation and esophageal distention. Ann Allergy 47:431-434
3. Kjellen G, Tibbling L, Wranne B (1981) Bronchial obstruction after oesophageal acid perfusion in asthmatic. Clin Physiol 1:285-292
4. Tan WC, Martin RJ, Pandy R, et al (1990) Effects of spontaneous and stimulated gastroesophaeal reflux on sleeping asthmatics. Am Rev Respir Dis 141:1394-1399
5. Schan CA, Harding SM, Haile JM, et al (1994) Gastroesophageal reflux-induced bronchoconstriction: an intraesophageal acid infusion study using state-of-the art technology. Chest 106:731-737
6. Harding SM, Guzzo MR, Maples R, et al (1995) Gastroesophageal reflux induced bronchoconstriction: vagolytic doses of atropine diminish airway responses to esophageal acid infusion. Am J Respir Crit Care Med 151:A589 (abstract)

7. Harding SM, Schan CA, Guzzo MR, et al (1995) Gastroesphageal reflux-induced bronchoconstriction: is microaspiration a factor? Chest 108:1220-1227

8. Jack CIA, Calverley PMA, Donnelly RJ, et al (1995) Simultaneous tracheal and oesophageal pH measurement in asthmatic patients with gastro-oesophageal reflux. Thorax 50:201-204

9. Ekstrom T, Tibbling L (1989) Esophageal acid perfusion, airway function, and symptoms in asthmatic patients with marked bronchial hyperreactivity. Chest 96:995-998

10. Herve P, Denjean A, Jian R, et al (1986) Intraesophageal perfusion of acid increases the bronchomotor response to methacholine and to isocapnic hyperventilation in asthmatic subjects. Am Rev Respir Dis 134:986-989

11. Wright RA, Miller SA, Corsello BF (1991) Acid-induced esophago-bronchial cardiac reflexes in humans. Gastroenterology 99:71-73

12. Holmes PW, Campbell AM, Barter CE (1975) Changes of lung volumes and lung mechanics in asthma and normal subjects. Thorax 33:394-400

13. Moote W, Lioyd DA, Mc Courtie DR (1986) Increase in gastroesophageal reflux during methacholine-induced bronchospasm. J Allergy Clin Immunol 78:619-623

14. Pomari C, Micheletto C, Dal Negro R (1997) MCH-induced broncho-constriction does not enhance gastro-esophageal reflux (GER). Eur Respir J 10(Suppl 25):58s

15. Pratter MR, Irwin RS (1984) The clinical value of pharmacologic bronchoprovocation challenge. Chest 85:260-66

16. Dal Negro R, Allegra L (1989) Blood gas changes during and after nonspecific airway challenge. J Appl Physiol 67:2627-2630

17. Pomari C, Micheletto C, Dal Negro R (1995) The UNDW-induced $PtcCO_2$ time-course of subjects with persistent cough due to GER proves peculiar. Am J Respir Crit Care Med 151:A412

18. Dal Negro RW, Turco P, Allegra L (1992) Blood gas exchanges in nonasthmatic rhinitics during and after nonspecific challenge. Am Rev Respir Dis 145:337-339

19. Pomari C, Micheletto C, Turco P, et al (1997) Acid drink enhances MCH response in GER only in subjects showing hypoxic response to UNDW. Eur Respir J 10:66s

20. Girelli-Bruni E, Tognella S, Dal Negro R (1996) Modelli di studio matematico-statistici. In: Dal Negro R (ed) Reattività bronchiale in salute e malattia. It J Chest Dis Publ, pp 55-54

21. Pomari C, Micheletto C, Dal Negro R (1996) UNDW-induced hyperventilation confirms as the peculiar hyperreactive feature in asymptomatic subjects with gastro-esophageal reflux (GER). Eur Respir J 9(Suppl 23):85-86

22. Lee BP, Sant'Ambrogio G, Sant'Ambrogio FB (1992) Different innervation and receptors of the canine extrathoracic trachea. Respir Physiol 90:55-65

23. Pomari C, Micheletto C, Dal Negro R (1996) Reattività bronchiale e reflusso gastro-esofageo. In: Dal Negro R (ed) Reattività bronchiale in salute e malattia. It J Chest Dis Publ, pp 55-58

24. Dal Negro R, Pomari C, Micheletto C, Turco P (1996) Omeprazole (OM), but not placebo (P), reduces the bronchial response to methacholine (MCH) in mild non-atopic asthmatics with gastroesophageal reflux (GER). Am J Respir Crit Care Med 153:A517

25. Dal Negro R, Pomari C, Turco P, Allegra L (1994) Gastroesophageal reflux and bronchial asthma: a cross over omeprazole vs placebo comparison. Am J Respir Crit Care Med 149:A202

26. Levin TR, Sperling RM, McQuaid KR (1998) Omeprazole improves peak expiratory flow rate and quality of life in asthmatics with gastroesophageal reflux. Am J Gastroenterol 93:1060-1063

27. Dal Negro R, Tognella S, Micheletto C, Turco P, Trevisan F, Pomari C (1998)

Pantoprazole 40 mg, but not placebo, improves the non-specific bronchial hyperresponsiveness in non atopic asthmatics with GER. Chest 114:297

28. Micheletto C, Burti E, Mauroner L, Pomari C, Turco P, Dal Negro R (1997) Induced sputum and serum inflammatory markers in subjects with cough due to gastroesophageal reflux. Eur Respir J 10(Suppl 25):317s

29. Micheletto C, Mauroner L, Burti E, Pomari C, Dal Negro R (1997) Induced sputum examination and serum inflammatory markers in asthma due to gastro-esophageal reflux. Eur Respir J 10(Suppl 25):317s

30. Venge P (1993) Serum measurements of eosinophil cationic protein (ECP) in bronchial asthma. Clin Exp Allergy 23:3-7

Fiberoptic Bronchoscopy and Bronchoalveolar Lavage in the Management of Children with Gastroesophageal Reflux

O. Sacco, B. Fregonese, M. Silvestri, and G.A. Rossi

Introduction

Patients with gastroesophageal reflux (GER) often show diffuse or localized esophagitis, characterized by esophageal mucosal damage resulting from reflux of gastric contents into the esophagus. This complication of GER is well characterized and is extensively described in all textbooks of internal medicine and pediatrics, whose authors postulate that reflux in the absence of esophagitis is usually asymptomatic [1-4]. In contrast, it is well accepted that gastric contents may reach the pharynx and mouth only during severe reflux episodes, resulting in laryngitis, morning hoarseness and recurrent pulmonary aspiration and leading to pulmonary infiltrates or chronic asthma [5-7]. The incidence of GER is high in pediatric patients and is mainly related to low esophageal sphincter (LES) tone [8]. In adults, GER incidence decreases and appears to be more frequently related to anatomical malposition of the viscera, as observed in the herniation of the stomach through the esophageal hiatus.

A variety of tests, such as esophageal pH recording, barium swallow, esophagoscopy with mucosal biopsy and esophageal motility evaluation, may be helpful to assess the presence and the severity of reflux, its pathophysiology, the nature of refluxant and the presence and the severity of the esophagitis [9-13]. These diagnostic procedures, however, do not give any information about the recurrence of pulmonary aspiration in GER patients: therefore in many patients the relationship between GER and respiratory symptoms can only be suspected on a clinical background. Even the "gold standard" diagnostic procedure, the long-term (24-hour) esophageal pH recording (pHmetry), which can suggest the occurrence of chronic aspiration in the presence of a severe GER, does not give any real proof. In addition, even when pHmetry is negative for clinically relevant GER, few or even a single reflux episode can induce aspiration of gastric contents, particularly if GER occurs during the sleeping hours.

Division of Pneumology, G. Gaslini Institute, Genoa, Italy

Gastroesophageal Reflux and the Respiratory Tract

As a consequence of the lack of tests to monitor and clinically study the aspiration of gastric contents in the airways, the pathophysiology of the respiratory symptoms associated with GER is not completely understood. Two major mechanisms that are not mutually exclusive have been proposed. The first is based on the direct soiling of the airways by acidic gastric fluid. This can occur as "macroaspiration" producing massive pulmonary infiltrates, as originally described by Mendelson [14] during the induction of obstetric anesthesia, or as "silent microaspiration". In the latter case, the irritant receptors in the trachea and airways are stimulated but the aspirated material is confined to the bronchial tree by the normal protective mechanisms: the offending aspirate is gradually removed by cough and mucociliary clearance before reaching the deep lung [14, 15].

The second proposed mechanism hypothesizes that the presence of acidic gastric juice in the distal esophagus stimulates mucosal esophageal receptors with the induction of vagal-mediated cough and bronchoconstriction. This indirect airway stimulation, which has been proven experimentally in both animals and humans, may indeed occur also in real life and explain why the presence of respiratory symptoms by itself is not enough to prove gastric aspiration.

Bronchoscopy in Patients with Gastroesophageal Reflux

Fiberoptic bronchoscopy, with direct visualization of the bronchial tree, is the only diagnostic procedure able to reveal whether the respiratory mucosa has recently been exposed to offending agents. However, endoscopy alone is not able to differentiate the mucosal inflammation due to chronic aspiration of gastric contents from that due to other causes, particularly in patients with a clinical history of chronic respiratory symptoms [16, 17]

Although there are no available tests which are both specific and sensitive for diagnosing chronic aspiration, the presence of lipid-laden macrophages (lipophages) in the airways has been reported to be strongly suggestive of food aspiration [18, 19]. Therefore, patients with GER and respiratory symptoms who undergo fiberoptic bronchoscopy as part of the diagnostic procedures should undergo at the same time bronchoalveolar lavage to evaluate the presence of lipophages and to characterize the degree and the cytological appearance of the bronchial inflammation.

A grading system for semiquantitating the amount of intracellular lipid in phagocytes ("lipid index") has been proposed by different authors. The amount of lipids per single macrophage may be evaluated by staining the cells with Nile red or oil red O and giving a score from 0 to 4 for each cell (Fig. 1). Score 0 indicates the absence of intracellular lipid droplets, while score 4 indicates the presence of many confluent intracellular droplets completely opacifying the cytoplasm and obscuring the nucleus. The final index is determined by evaluating 100 cells; 400 is the highest possible score [19].

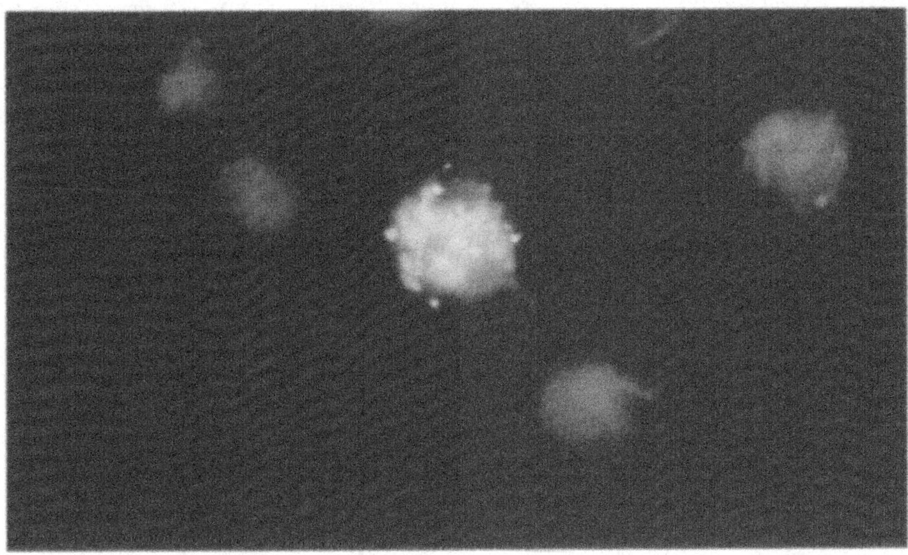

Fig. 1. Cytospin preparation of bronchoalveolar lavage cells evaluated by fluorescence microscopy, demonstrating the presence of one lipid-laden macrophage (Nile red oil staining, original magnification x 1000) surrounded by Nile red-negative cells

Although the grading procedure is quite simple by itself, some problems may arise. First, lipophages can be present in a variety of respiratory disorders other than those induced by GER. Indeed, Nile red and oil red O stains are not specific for exogenous lipids, since they also enhance endogenous lipids resulting from local tissue breakdown. Therefore, lipid-laden alveolar macrophages may be recovered during acute lung injury and recurrent or chronic respiratory diseases, such as obstructive pneumonia. Second, small amounts of intracellular lipids may be found in a low proportion of macrophages obtained from normal controls. Third, the presence of lipophages in the lavage fluid adds by itself little information about the origin of the aspirate. Actually, the aspirate may result from dysphagia (aspiration from above), quite common in neurologically impaired patients, rather than from GER (aspiration from below).

To overcome these problems, studies were performed to set different cut-off values for the lipid index. The wide range of lipid-laden macrophage indexes tested by probability statistics showed that as the value of the cut-off between "aspirator" and "nonaspirator" patients was increased, the test became more specific but less sensitive. On the contrary, as the cut-off was reduced, test sensitivity increased but specificity decreased. There is now consensus about the usefulness of this laboratory test as a screening between aspirator and nonaspirator patients, but probably the best lipid index cut-off to differentiate these two groups of patients should change in different patient populations (i.e. patients with or without neurological problems or adult versus pediatric patients). The lipid index cut-off most often used in adults (> 70 or 100) is probably not suited as a screening for aspirators among children. Another bias in the literature is due to inhomogeneous study populations that include patients with parenchymal lung disease not clearly related to aspiration of gastric contents and not well-characterized on the presence or absence of GER [19-20].

Bronchoscopy and Bronchoalveolar Lavage in Children with Gastroesophageal Reflux

In the pediatric population, GER is quite common and frequently associated with respiratory symptoms usually not responding to the standard respiratory therapy. These include laryngospasm, recurrent infections, and chronic/recurrent asthma-like symptoms. Pediatric patients with respiratory symptoms and a clinical history suggesting GER are usually evaluated by 24-hour esophageal pH monitoring (pHmetry) as a first-line diagnostic procedure. The presence of peptic esophagitis must be evaluated by esophagoscopy when pHmetry suggests severe GER. This may occur when the esophageal pH is < 4 in more than 4% of the recorded time, when there is a high number of episodes of pH < 4, or when there is a high number of episodes of pH < 4 lasting longer than 5 min [2, 9-11].

Fiberoptic bronchoscopy (with bronchoalveolar lavage) may be performed in these "severe GER" patients at the same time as esophagoscopy. Bronchoscopy may also be indicated in neurologically normal individuals without dysphagia, when the clinical symptoms are suggestive for GER but pHmetry does not support this suspicion. Following these indications, we have recently performed fiberoptic bronchoscopy and bronchoalveolar lavage (BAL) in: (a) a group of "severe GER" children presenting recurrent respiratory symptoms, and (b) a group of clinically GER-positive children with negative pHmetry ("negative pHmetry" group). In these two patient groups, we evaluated: (a) the degree of airway inflammation by counting the number of BAL neutrophils, with an arbitrary cut-off of ≥ 5% between normal and pathological values; (b) the lipid index (LI), with an arbitrary cut-off of ≥ 20 discriminating scores considered suggestive or not suggestive for aspiration.

Among the severe GER patients, 57% had elevated BAL neutrophil counts and high LI, while 43% showed BAL neutrophil counts within the normal range and low LI. Among the negative pHmetry patients, only 29% had high BAL neutrophil counts and a high LI (Fig. 2). In both groups, an elevated LI was always associated with high BAL neutrophil counts, suggesting that airway neutrophilia, at least in pediatric patients, may be considered a secondary index of gastric aspiration. Finally, in the severe GER patients, there were no correlations between the severity of GER and LI scores or BAL neutrophilia.

With the combined analysis of BAL and pHmetry data, it was possible to divide GER patients into the following four groups: (a) patients with positive pHmetry, high BAL neutrophils and high LI (i.e. patients with severe GER, leading to aspiration and gastric contents reaching the deep lung); (b) patients with

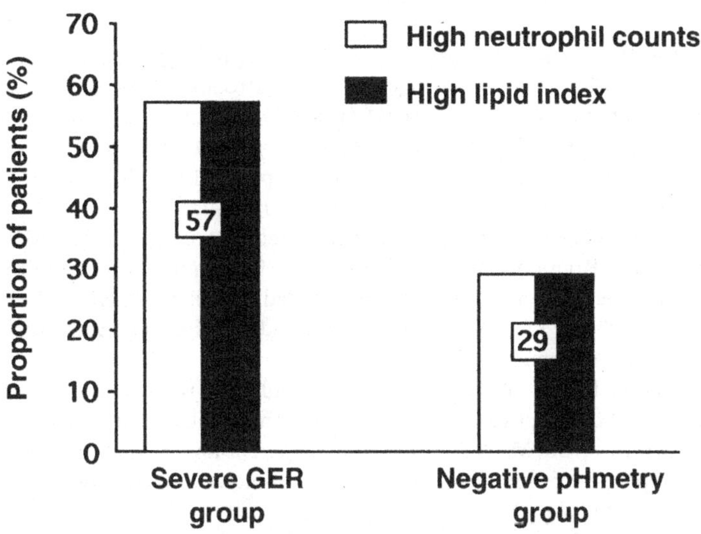

Fig. 2. Proportion of patients with high lipid index (LI) and elevated neutrophil counts in children with GER and recurrent respiratory problems (*severe GER group*) or in clinically GER-positive children with negative pHmetry (*negative pHmetry group*)

positive pHmetry but with normal BAL neutrophils and low LI (i.e. patients with GER but without clinically relevant gastric aspiration); (c) patients with negative pHmetry but with high BAL neutrophil counts and high LI (i.e. patients with infrequent, but clinically relevant GER episodes, not fully detected by pHmetry); and (d) patients with negative pHmetry, normal BAL neutrophil counts and low LI (patients with respiratory symptoms not related to reflux or with rare episodes of GER, without direct soiling of the airways by gastric contents).

Conclusions

From these observations, we conclude that patients with respiratory symptoms and a clinical history suggesting GER do not form a homogeneous group, and that pHmetry data alone do not satisfactorily describe the different clinical pictures. BAL and pHmetry are two complementary diagnostic procedures whose data, when considered together, are particularly helpful in evaluating the presence of gastric content inhalation. Because these procedures are both relatively invasive, they should be performed only in selected patient groups, at least in the pediatric population.

Acknowledgements. Supported by Ricerca Corrente 1994, Ministero della Sanità, Rome, Italy.

References

1. Fisher RB, Marmud LS, Robert GS, Lobis IF (1976) Gastroesophageal scintiscanning to detect and quantitate gastroesophageal reflux. Gastroenterology 70:301-308
2. Boix-Ochoa J, Lefunte JM, Gill-Vernet JM (1980) Twentyfour hour esophageal pH-monitoring in gastroesophageal reflux. J Pediatr Surg 15:74-78
3. Euler AR, Byrne WJ (1981) Twentyfour hour esophageal intraluminal pH probe testing: a comparative analysis. Gastroenterology 80:957-961
4. Carré IJ (1985) Management of gastroesophageal reflux. Arch Dis Child 60:71-75
5. Hoyoux C, Forget P, Lambrech L, Geubelle F (1985) Chronic bronchopulmonary disease and gastroesophageal reflux in children. Pediatr Pulmonol 1:149-153
6. Herbst JJ, Book LS, Bry PF (1978) Gastroesophageal reflux in the "near miss" sudden infant death syndrome. J Pediatr 92:73-75
7. Danus O, Casar C, Labrain A, Pope CE (1976) Esophageal reflux and unrecognized cause of recurrent obstructive bronchitis in children. J Pediatr 89:220-224
8. Cristhie DL, O'Grady LR, Mack DV (1978) Incompetent lower esophageal sphincter and gastroesophageal reflux in recurrent acute pulmonary disease of infancy and childood. J Pediatr 93:23-27
9. Cucchiara S, Staiano L, Gobio-Casati L, et al (1988) La pHmetria intraesofagea prolungata nella diagnosi della malattia da reflusso gastroesofageo. Riv Ital Ped 14:187-195
10. Da Dalt L, Mazzoleni S, Montini G, Donzelli F, Zacchello F (1989) Diagnostic accuracy of pH monitoring in gastroesophageal reflux. Arch Dis Child 64:1421-1426
11. Vandenplas Y, Sacré L, Loeb H (1989) pH monitoring in children. Neth J Med 34:562-573
12. Reich SD, Early WC, Goodman M, Spector S, Stein MR (1977) Evaluation of gastropulmonary aspiration by a radioactive technique. J Nucl Med 18:1079-1081
13. Gustavson IN, Kjelman NI, Tibbling L (1986) Oesophageal function and symptoms in moderate and severe asthma. Acta Pediatr Scand 5:729-733
14. Mendelson CL (1964) The aspiration of stomach contents into the lungs during obstetric anesthesia. Am J Obstet Gynecol 52:191-204
15. Taussing LM, Lemen RJ (1979) Chronic obstructive lung disease. Adv Pediatr 26:343-416
16. Rossi GA (1986) Bronchoalveolar lavage in the investigation of disorders of the lower respiratory tract. Eur J Respir Dis 69:293-315
17. Reynolds HY (1987) Bronchoalveolar lavage. Am Rev Respir Dis 135:250-263
18. Williams HE, Freeman M (1973) Milk inhalation pneumonia, the significance of fat filled macrophages in tracheal secretion. Aust Paediatr J 9:286-288
19. Colombo JL, Timothy KH (1987) Recurrent aspiration in children: lipid-laden alveolar macrophage quantitation. Pediatr Pulmonol 3:86-89
20. Nussbaum E, Maggi JC, Mathis R, Galant SP (1987) Association of lipid-laden alveolar macrophages and gastroesophageal reflux in children. J Pediatr 110:190-194

Therapy

Therapy of Gastroesophageal Reflux Disease: The Gastroenterological Approach

L. Okolicsanyi and C. Guatti-Zuliani

Introduction

Gastroesophageal reflux disease (GERD), the most common disorder of the esophagus, is extremely variable in its presentations and clinical course. It is known from epidemiological studies that many people complain of typical reflux symptoms, including heartburn and regurgitation, but only few request medical investigation. About 20%-40% of the world's population has symptoms suggestive of GERD; an exact estimate is difficult because of the way the disease presents [1]. In 1985, Castell [2] described GERD as an iceberg, with a large base indicating patients with slight and episodic symptoms without need of medical assistance, a smaller portion of patients with moderate and recurrent symptoms and, at the top, patients with severe and persistent symptoms requiring special care (Fig. 1). Furthermore, a number of patients with atypical symptoms, such as refractory asthma, recurrent hoarseness, chronic unexplained cough or non-cardiac chest pain, are later discovered as having GERD. Thus, it seems evident that this disease is frequently underdiagnosed.

GERD not only represents a common and costly condition with an erratic course, but also is relevant because of severe complications, including peptic ulcer, secondary strictures, Barrett's esophagus and ultimately adenocarcinoma. Early recognition of the disease and correct therapeutic procedures are able to control symptoms and prevent complications.

Pathophysiology

Under physiological conditions, anatomic and functional elements together assure an antireflux barrier between the esophagus and the stomach (Table 1) [3]. Acid reflux from stomach to esophagus is a physiological phenomenon which occurs many times in a day, particularly during the post-prandial period.

Gastroenterology Section, Institute of Medical Semeiology, University of Parma, Italy

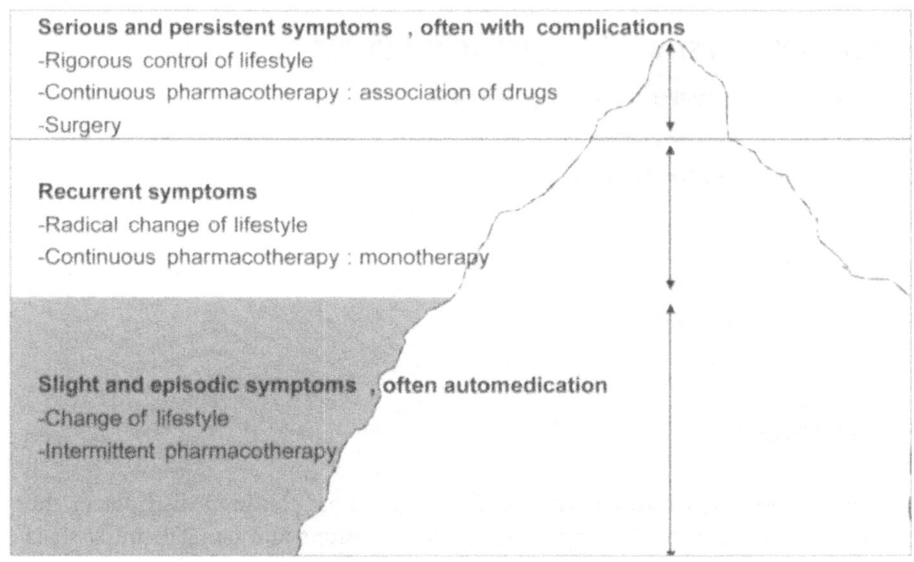

Fig. 1. The iceberg of patients with GERD. (Modified from [2])

Table 1. Anatomic and functional elements of antireflux barrier

Extrinsic compression of LES by diaphragmatic crura
Presence of an intra-abdominal segment of esophagus
Integrity of phreno-esophageal ligament
Angle of His
Motility pattern of LES

LES, lower esophageal sphincter

However, when it happens too often and in excessive measures, manifest symptoms and anatomic lesions may appear.

GERD is primarily a motility disorder of the esophagus and stomach with impaired capacity of clearing and decreased lower esophageal sphincter (LES) pressure. Transient LES relaxation appears to be the most important mechanism of reflux [4]. Table 2 shows the detailed pathogenetic mechanisms of GERD.

Incompetence of Anti-Reflux Barrier

Anatomically the diaphragmatic channel and the intra-abdominal segment of esophagus, functionally the LES, are the major elements of the barrier [5]. In GERD normal or low pressure of LES is seen, but transient LES relaxation appears to be the most important mechanism of reflux. Reflux is a swallow-independent relaxation during which the pressure decreases and reaches the gastric pressure for at least 5 s [6-8].

Table 2. Major factors in the pathogenesis of GERD

Incompetence of anti-reflux barrier
Deficit of esophageal clearance
Deficit of mucosal resistance
Potency of refluxate to cause injury
Concomitant factors: hiatus hernia and delayed gastric emptying
Helicobacter pylori
Esophageal hypersensitivity

Impairment of Esophageal Clearance

In physiological conditions, three factors are important for the efficacy of the esophageal clearance mechanism: gravity, peristaltic esophageal motor activity and capacity of saliva in neutralizing residual amounts of acid. However, in GERD non-peristaltic contractions and reduced saliva production are currently found [9-11].

Altered Mucosal Resistence

The mucosal resistence is made by mucus, bicarbonate ions, an unstirred water layer on the epithelial cells, the presence of tight intercellular junctions, and elevated cell replication and vascularization. Acid exposure may lead to variable degrees of mucosal damage if some of these components are impaired [11].

Potency of Refluxate to Cause Injury

Acid is the most important element in the development of damage, even if in GERD there is usually not an increase of acid secretion at baseline or after a meal. The action of acid in injury may also involve pepsin activation. It is unclear whether bile acids can induce damage by themselves or by amplifying the destructive power of hydrogen ions [12].

Hiatus Hernia

A direct causal relationship does not seem to exist. Nevertheless, a hiatus hernia may interfere with normal esophageal clearance [13]

Delayed Gastric Emptying

This causes gastric distention post-prandially that increases reflux and the rate of transient LES relaxation [14].

Role of *Helicobacter pylori*

The relation between *H. pylori* and GERD remains controversial. Recently, Labenz et al. [15] suggested a protective role of *H. pylori* on GERD: incidence of reflux esophagitis within three years after *H. pylori* eradication to cure duodenal ulcer disease was 26%, compared to 13% in individuals in whom the infection persisted. However, this intriguing observation is not easily explained.

Esophageal Hypersensitivity

Most episodes of reflux are not perceived by patients [16]. Some factors are known to contribute to this perception, for example, the duration of reflux episodes or the length of acid exposure [17]; however, there are large inter- and intra-individual variations. Twenty-four hour pH monitoring (pHmetry) studies enabled the identification of a group of subjects with hypersensitivity to acid exposure. In this group, there was a clear-cut correlation between episodes of reflux and symptoms [18]. The same subjects were also highly sensitive to mechanical stimuli such as balloon distension. Chemical and mechanical receptors located in the esophageal wall are mostly responsible for this hypersensitivity. It can also explain the relationship between esophagus and heart and lung: a vagally mediated reflex can provoke bronchial constriction and chronic repetitive throat clearing and coughing in patients with GERD [19].

Medical Therapy

General Measures

Tables 3 and 4 show the lifestyle and hygienic-dietetic measures to be adopted by patients with GERD. In fact, these are the cornerstone of effective antireflux treatment: there are no definite results of medical therapy without careful acceptance of these recommendations. Some sample maneuvers will produce immediate results, such as avoiding increases of intra-abdominal pressure. Elevation of the head of the bed is a simple, inexpensive and effective device for GERD. It improves acid clearance time, reduces esophageal exposure to acid [20], and is particularly useful when associated with H_2 receptor blocker administration [21]. An alternative procedure is the use of a firm wedge; using several pillows should be avoided, because it is painful to the neck and does not provide stable support throughout the night (the patient easily rolls off while asleep).

Table 3. Therapeutic approach to GERD: lifestyle measures

- Avoid what increases intra-abdominal pressure: weight gain, sports with elevated abdominal muscle contraction, tight clothing
- Avoid bending of trunk
- Do not lie down immediately after meals
- Avoid meals and drinking 2-3 hours before retiring
- Elevate head of bed of about 15-20 cm
- Lie preferably on the left side

Table 4. Therapeutic approach to GERD: hygienic-dietetic measures

Small and frequent meals
Avoid
   Excessive meals
   Foods that reduce LES pressure
   Irritating foods
   Foods that delay gastric emptying
   Alcohol
Stop smoking
Attention to concomitant medication

Meals should be small and taken frequently, and should not contain particular foods that reduce LES pressure like chocolate, fat, onion, mint and carminatives. Foods irritating the esophageal mucosa should also be abandoned: these are alcohol drinks, coffee, fruit and tomato juices. Low-fat meals reduce gastric volume and are also useful for caloric control. Slight weight loss may drammatically improve reflux symptoms [22]. Smoking should be stopped, because it reduces LES pressure and prolongs acid exposure [23].

The reevaluation of concomitant drugs is relevant, since many compounds may have direct harmful effects on the esophagogastric mucosa and may also decrease LES pressure (Table 5). In elderly, obese individuals with GERD, the use of non-steroid anti-inflammatory drugs (NSAIDs) must be avoided.

Table 5. Drugs that contribute to GERD

Agents that decrease LES pressure
   Benzodiazepines
   Calcium channel blockers
   Theophylline
   β-Adrenergic agonists
   α-Adrenergic antagonist
   Meperidine
   Anticholinergic agents
   Tricyclic antidepressants
   Progesterone

Agents that injure the esophageal mucosa
   NSAIDs
   Iron salts
   Slow release KCl
   Tetracycline
   Doxycycline
   Quinidine

NSAIDs, non-steroid anti-inflammatory drugs

Medical Approach

The specific aims of medical therapy are first of all, to enhance quality of life [24-27] by releaving symptoms, healing esophagitis when present (in Table 6

Table 6. Savary-Miller classification of reflux esophagitis

Grade	Endoscopic findings
I	Nonconfluent erythematous lesions proximal to the mucosal junction
II	Confluent, noncircumferential erosive exudative lesions
III	Circumferential, confluent erythematous areas and erosions
IV	Complicated esophagitis: deep ulcer or stricture formation

the endoscoping grading is presented), and by preventing further complications (e.g. strictures, Barrett's metaplasia). Furthermore, control of relapses and maintenance of remission are mandatory.

Initially, in patients without endoscopically demonstrated signs of esophagitis and with mild to moderate symptomatic reflux disease, antacids are useful. Intermediate cases without manifest signs of esophagitis, but with more intense symptoms may respond to full-dose H_2 receptor blocker treatment. The association with prokinetic drugs is considered to be optional (favorable in our own experience). When the patient does not respond to this therapy or when inflammatory lesions of the esophagus are found, more intense drug therapy is requested. It consists in full-dose employment of proton pump inhibitors (PPIs) given in divided doses for a minimum of three months [28,29]. Even if the patient's symptoms and esophagitis resolve, maintenance therapy should be taken into account, since in about 50% of cases, specific symptoms relapse a few months after complete remission [30-32]. Maintenance therapy can be continuous or discontinuous for 2-4 weeks, the latter being better accepted by patients and having a favorable cost-benefit ratio [33,34]. In Table 7, the doses of PPIs most frequently used for GERD and esophagitis are summarized.

A small portion of individuals (no more than 5% reported in the literature) fails medical treatment. For these cases presenting medically intractable symptoms and complications, a surgical antireflux procedure is requested [35,36]. Nissen fundoplication is the most frequently employed procedure [37].

Table 8 shows the main objectives of medical therapy. These are mostly directed to re-establishing physiological conditions whenever possible, by decreasing eccessive acid secretion and increasing resting LES pressure. The improvement of esophageal motor function and acid clearence is essential in this procedure.

Drug Therapy

The main pharmacological agents effective in GERD therapy are reported in Table 9.

Antacids

These drugs, the most widely used compounds for treatment of heartburn, are most frequently purchased by patients in the drug store. Antacids work by neutralizing gastric acid and by increasing intragastric pH, albeit for a relatively

Table 7. Medical treatment of GERD + esophagitis: use of PPIs

Drug	Indication	Dose
Omeprazole	Acute therapy	20-40 mg/day, 4-8 weeks
	Maintenance therapy	20 mg/day
Lansoprazole	Acute therapy	30 mg/day, 4-8 weeks
	Maintenance therapy	15 mg/day
Pantoprazole	Acute therapy	40 mg/day, < 8 weeks
	Maintenance therapy	20 mg/day

Table 8. Therapeutic approach to GERD: main objectives

Decrease gastric secretion
Increase resting LES pressure
Enhance gastric emptying
Make esophageal refluxate innocuous
Improve esophageal motor function
Enhance esophageal acid clearance
Stimulate salivation
Improve esophageal protection
Promote esophageal healing

Table 9. Therapeutic approach to GERD: drug therapy

Antacids
   Aluminium/magnesium hydroxide

Prokinetic agents
   Metoclopramide
   Domperidone
   Levosulpiride
   Cisapride

Cytoprotective and barrier drugs
   Carbenoxolone
   Prostaglandins
   Sucralfate
   Alginic acid

Antisecretive agents
   H_2-antagonists
   Proton pump inhibitors

short period of time. They appear to be effective in controlling mild to moderate symptoms, but administration should be frequent (3-4 times daily). The best results are seen when antacids are taken 30-60 min after meals and at bedtime [38,39]. Their effect is usually transitory in individuals without esophagitis. Often, side effects such as diarrhea or chronic constipation develop.

Prokinetic Agents

These drugs are used for the treatment of reflux disease because they increase LES pressure, enhance gastric emptying, and improve esphageal peristaltic function [40]. Metoclopramide is a benzamide derivative that acts as a dopamine antagonist and cholinergic agonist [41]. It increases LES pressure and gastric peristalsis and consequently facilitates gastric emptying [42] and removes the stimulus of vomiting; this drug has no effect on gastric acid secretion [43-45]. The most important side effects are fatigue, lethargy, and psychotropic and extrapyramidal concerns, all of which are reversible on cessation of drug therapy, although tardive dyskinesia may persist. The dopamine-antagonistic property of metoclopramide may also lead to hyperprolactinemia and galactorrhea, which can be avoided by decreasing the daily dose or by giving the drug only before a large meal.

Domperidone is a dopamine-receptor antagonist which also increases gastrointestinal motility and LES pressure [46]. It rarely has central nervous system (CNS) side effects because it crosses the blood-brain barrier poorly. The usual dosage is 20 mg taken 15-30 min before meals and before bedtime. Side effects, which occur in a reduced portion of patients, are headaches, diarrhea and anxiety. More rarely, dystonic and extrapyramidal signs are seen. Hyperprolactinemia with breast enlargement, galactorrhea and amenorrhea may also occur.

Levosulpride acts on presynaptic and postsynaptic dopaminergic receptors in the submucosal and myoenteric plexus. Its effect are both central (anti-hemetic and neuroleptic) and peripheral. At low doses it has a synergic effect with acetylcholine: it favors gastric emptying and increases the resting LES pressure [47]. Undesired side effects are insomnia, extrapyramidal symptoms and hyperprolactinemia with related symptoms.

Cisapride, a substituted piperidinyl benzamide, stimulates acetylcholine release in the myenteric plexus of the upper gastrointestinal tract, thus raising esophageal sphincter pressure and gut motility [48-50]. 5-HT$_3$ receptor antagonism and 5-HT$_4$ receptor agonism may also play major roles in its mode of action [51]. Cisapride is not an antidopaminergic agent and does not cross the blood-brain barrier. It has no effect on acid secretion, while it increases salivary and esophageal secretions, thus favoring esophageal acid clearance and mucosal resistence [8]. Rare side effects consist in diarrhea, abdominal cramps and tachycardia.

Cytoprotective and Barrier Drugs

Sucralfate is a complex salt of aluminum and sucrose octa-sulfate. It releases aluminum ions on exposure to acid, producing negatively charged molecules that bind tightly to positively charged necrotic ulcer tissue, thus forming a physical barrier to prevent further injury [39]. Sucralfate may also stimulate local production of endogenous prostaglandins and growth factors [52-54]. It does not suppress gastric acid secretion, but reduces the absorption of a number of other orally administered drugs (e.g. antibiotics, theophylline, digoxin)

[55]. Few unwanted side effects are constipation, nausea, headache and rashes.

Alginic acid, often taken in association with antacids, is commonly used for heartburn. Alginic acid reacts with saliva to form a highly viscous solution that floats on the surface of the gastric pool, acting as a mechanical barrier which can reduce the number of reflux episodes and diminish esophageal acid exposure. It is a weak antacid, does not change gastric pH [39], and has no effect on LES pressure. It is usefully employed in mild forms of GERD, although it is not better than commonly used antacids [56-58].

Antisecretive Agents

H_2 Antagonists. These agents exert substantial effects in the treatment of symptomatic GERD. However, their efficacy in healing esophagitis is not as evident as that found in healing peptic ulcer [59-61]. These drugs have no effect on LES pressure nor on esophageal or gastric motility. Their only known mechanism of action is decreasing gastric acid production. These agents are equally effective when employed in proper doses [62].

Cimetidine, the first commercially available H_2 blocker, is still available but less commonly used because of antiandrogenic side effects [63] and competition with intrahepatic metabolism of several frequently employed benzodiazepines, theophylline or anticoagulants [64].

Ranitidine is a strong gastric acid suppressor, is safely used because it does not interfere with hepatic drug metabolism, and is normally metabolized in aged patients. It is the first choice drug in mild to medium forms of GERD. Doses of 150 mg are generally administered twice daily and at bedtime for maintenance therapy [65]. Recently, it was seen that lower doses (75 mg at bed-time) are particularly useful in preventing symptom relapses. Ranitidine is also available in soluble preparations. The incidence of side effects is about 5% or less. Headache and dizziness are among the most commonly reported side effects. More rarely, a variety of apparently idiosyncratic reactions have been reported, including fever, hematological and liver disorders, nephritis and cardiac arrhythmias.

Famotidine, nizatidine and roxatidine (the newest of the H_2 receptor antagonists) are also available, even if they are less commonly used in clinical practice. According to recent studies, roxatidine, more than other H_2 blockers, stimulated growth factors and ulcer healing.

Proton Pump Inhibitors. There is now increasing clinical evidence about the superiority of proton pump inhibitors (PPIs) over standard dose H_2 receptor antagonists in GERD treatment. The most important data come from a recent meta-analysis pooling 43 studies, including more than 7000 patients with esophagitis and GERD [66]. In this study, it was clearly demonstrated that a significantly higher proportion of patients was healed and rendered asymptomatic with PPIs, when compared to individuals treated with H_2 blockers (84% vs. 52% healed and 77% vs. 48% symptom-free, respectively, Table 10) [66].

Table 10. Effect of H_2-receptor antagonists and PPIs on symptoms and healing of reflux esophagitis: meta-analysis of 43 studies. (Modified from [66])

	H_2-receptor antagonists (%)	PPIs (%)
Healed	52 ± 17	84 ± 11
Symptom-free	48 ± 15	77 ± 10
Healing rate	5.9	11.7
Relief rate	6.4	11.5

The first commercially available PPI was omeprazole [67]. Recently, the family of PPIs has grown with the presentation of other agents, such as lansoprazole and pantoprazole. These compounds are potent and long-acting inhibitors of both basal and stimulated gastric acid secretion. They act by selective non-competitive inhibition of the H^+/K^+ATPase enzyme activity, the so-called proton pump located in the secretory membrane of the gastric parietal cell (Fig. 2). The exchange of H^+ and K^+ by this pump is the final common pathway in acid secretion. Thus, proton pump inhibition reduces acid secretion stimulated by any means [68]. PPIs have no effect on LES pressure.

Omeprazole and lansoprazole have similar mechanisms of action. Both are benzimidazole sulfoxide prodrugs that are highly labile in acid. They are protected in the stomach in acid-resistant capsules which dissolve in the duodenum and upper jejunum. Actually, omeprazole i.v. is also available; it is useful when oral administration is not possible or in case of bleeding. Proton pump inhibitors reduce 24-hour acid secretion by more than 90%, compared with 50%-80% with standard doses of H_2-receptor antagonists. The long duration of action despite their short elimination half-life (about 2 h), is due to the time required for new pumps to be synthesized and inserted into the secretory membrane. Lansoprazole is about 25% more potent than omeprazole in humans [69]. Thus, a dose of 15 mg is comparable in antisecretory effect to 20 mg omeprazole [70, 71].

The important reduction of gastric acid secretion is not without risk. It stimulates gastrin release which promotes the proliferation of enterochromaffin-like cells in the gastric antrum [72]. In rats, but not in mice, there is experimental evidence about the development of carcinoid tumors in relation to high levels of serum gastrin [73].

In man, short-term treatment with PPIs is safe and without side effects. Gastrin levels usually rise to values only 2-3 times above normal, and remain at this level during long-term therapy for up to 18 months. With discontinuation of the drug, gastrin levels return to normal. However, in a small subset of patients, serum gastrin levels may rise to elevated values (more than 1000 pg/ml). Usually, these changes are present during the first eight weeks of therapy [74-76].

There is still debate about later consequences of prolonged PPI treatment in patients with associated chronic gastritis. The prolonged inhibition of gastric acid secretion may lead to atrophic gastritis. This has been observed after omepra-

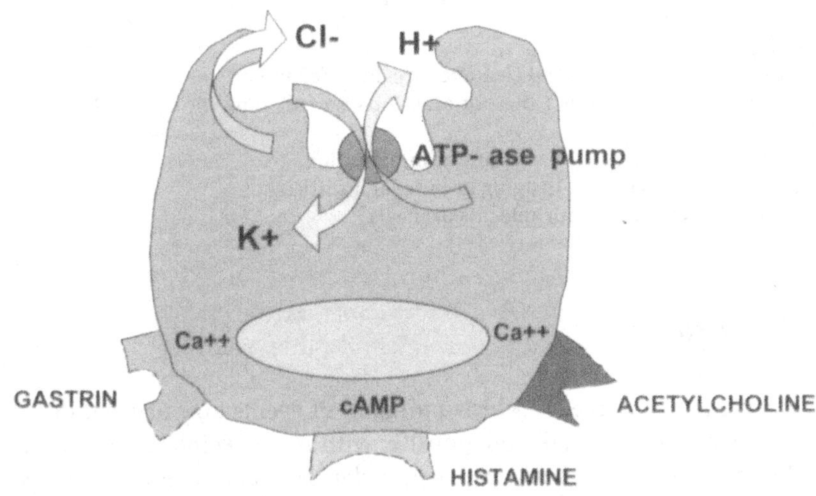

Fig. 2. The physiology of the hydrochloric acid secretory process

zole administration in *H. pylori*-positive patients, but was not confirmed in other studies [77-79]. The association of *H. pylori* and gastric cancer may further raise some doubts about prolonged PPI treatment: in fact, the question will require appropriate prospective, randomized studies for a definitive solution.

PPIs may interfere with cytochrome P450 enzyme activities, thus influencing the disposition of a series of xenobiotics, including warfarin, phenytoin, diazepam and prednisone [80]. It seems increasingly evident from the common clinical practice that these are not practically relevant interactions.

Pantoprazole [81] is the newest member of the PPI family, whose main pharmacokinetic characteristics are summarized in Table 11. It presents a rapid proton pump inhibitory action and has stronger pH stability and proton pump linkage specificity than omeprazole and lansoprazole [82-85]. No clinically relevant side effects are seen. In particular, there are few, if any, reports in the literature concerning interactions of pantoprazole with the metabolism of other drugs [86,87]. As far as its efficacy in GERD, a number of studies indicate that 40 mg daily administration in short- and medium-term treatments is as efficacious as omeprazole treatment (20 mg) [88, 89]. The same was observed in several comparative studies in patients with more severe forms of esophagitis (grades II and III) [90].

Finally, long-term maintenance studies carried out in Italy and in several other countries indicate that pantoprazole is able, like other PPIs, to prevent recurrences of esophagitis without evident side effects [91-93].

Table 11. Pharmacokinetic characteristics of pantoprazole

- $T_{1/2} = 1$ hour
- Distributive volume, half-life and clearance are dose-dependent
- Same pharmacokinetics after 1 dose or after 7 days of therapy (no accumulation of the drug)
- Low interindividual variations after oral administration
- No pharmacokinetic changes in aging or in renal insufficiency
- No absorbing interference with antacids or meals

Future Research

GERD is a complex disease for which a number of events may play pathogenetic roles [94-96]. Among these, the relationship with *H. pylori* infection is not completely known [79, 97, 98]. It seems that *H. pylori* is not an important risk factor for GERD. On the contrary, it appears a weakly protective one [15, 99]. Therefore, eradication therapy in diagnosed patients is not mandatory before long-term PPI treatment.

Future directions for research include the prevention of GERD in high-risk patients (obese, alcoholics, smokers, drug abusers, or individuals using drugs interferring with esophageal motility) and the development of specific therapies that reduce the rate of occurrence of transient LES relaxations [100]. These are the starting points for the symptomatic manifestations of GERD.

References

1. Spechler SJ (1992) Epidemiology and natural history of gastro-oesophageal reflux disease. Digestion 51(Suppl 1):24-29
2. Castell DO (1985) Introduction to pathophysiology of gastroesophageal reflux. In: Castell DO, Wu WC, Ott DJ (eds) Gastro-esophageal reflux disease. Futura, New York, pp 3-9
3. Mittal RK (1990) Current concepts of the antireflux barrier in gastroesophageal reflux disease. Gastroenterol Clin North Am 19:501-506
4. Mittal RK, McCallum RW (1988) Characteristics and frequency of transient relaxations of the lower esophageal sphincter in patients with reflux esophagitis. Gastroenterology 96:593-599
5. Zaninotto G, DeMeester TR, Schwiter W (1988) The lower esophageal sphincter in health and disease. Am J Surg 155:104-111
6. Dent J, Holloway RH, Toouli J, Dodds WJ (1988) Mechanisms of lower esophageal sphincter incompetence in patients with symptomatic gastro-esophageal reflux. Gut 29:1020-1028
7. Mittal RK, Holloway RH, Penagini R, Blackshaw LA, Dent J (1995) Transient lower esophageal sphincter relaxation. Gastroenterology 109:601-610
8. Dent J (1998) Gastro-oesophageal reflux disease. Digestion 59:433-445
9. Kahrilas PJ, Dodds WJ, Hogan WJ, Kern M, Arndorfer RC, Reece A (1986) Esophageal peristaltic dysfunction in peptic esophagitis. Gastroenterology 91:897-904

10. Helm JF, Dodds WJ, Pelc LR, Palmer DW, Hogan WJ, Teeter BC (1984) Effect of esophageal emptying and saliva on clearance of acid from esophagus. N Engl J Med 310:284-288

11. Orlando RC (1986) Esophageal epithelial resistance. J Clin Gastroenterol (8 Suppl) 1:12-16

12. Vaezi MF, Singh S, Richter JE (1995) Role of acid and duodenogastric reflux in oesophageal mucosal injury: a review of animal and human studies. Gastroenterology 108:1897-1907

13. Mittal RK, Lange RC, McCallum RW (1987) Identification and mechanism of delayed esophageal acid clearance in subjects with hiatus hernia. Gastroenterology 92:130-135

14. McCallum RW, Berkowitz BM, Lerner E (1981) Gastric emptying in patients with gastroesophageal reflux. Gastroenterology 80:285-291

15. Labenz J, Blum AL, Bayerdorffer E, Meining A, Stolte M, Börsch G (1997) Curing *Helicobacter* infection in patients with duodenal ulcer may provoke reflux oesophagitis. Gastroenterology 112:1442-1447

16. Baldi F, Ferrarini F, Longanesi A, Ragazzini M, Barbara L (1989) Acid gastro-oesophageal reflux and symptoms occurence. Analysis of some factors influencing their association. Dig Dis Sci 34:1890-1893

17. Galmiche JP, Scarpignato C (1995) Oesophageal sensitivity to acid in patients with non-cardiac chest pain: is the oesophagus hypersensitive? Eur J Gastroenterol Hepatol 7:1152-1159

18. Shi G, Bruley des Varannes S, Scarpignato C, Le Rhun M, Galmiche JP (1995) Reflux related symptoms in patients with normal oesophageal exposure to acid. Gut 37:457-464

19. Goldman J, Bennett JR (1988) Gastroesophageal disease and respiratory disorders in adults. Lancet ii:493-497

20. Johnson LF, DeMeester TR (1981) Evaluation of elevation of the bed, bethanechol and antiacid foam tablets on gastroesophageal reflux. Dig Dis Sci 26:673-680

21. Harvey RF, Gordon PC, Hadley N, et al (1987) Effect of sleeping with the bed-head raised and of ranitidine in patients with severe peptic esophagitis. Lancet ii:1200-1203

22. Dent J (1992) Long term aim of treatment of reflux disease and the role of non-drug measures. Digestion 51(Suppl 1):330-334

23. Kahrilas PJ, Gupta RR (1990) Mechanisms of acid reflux associated with cigarette smoking. Gut 31:4-10

24. Hunt RH (1993) Quality of life - the challenges ahead. Scand J Gastroenterol Suppl 199:2-4

25. Dimenäs E (1993) Methodological aspects of evalutation of quality of life in upper gastrointestinal diseases. Scand J Gastroenterol Suppl 199:18-21

26. Wilhelmsen I (1995) Quality of life in upper gastrointestinal disorders. Scand J Gastroenterol Suppl 211:21-25

27. Irvine EJ (1996) Measuring quality of life: a review. Scand J Gastroenterol Suppl 221:5-7

28. Vantrappen G, Rutgers L, Schurmans P, Coengrachts JL (1988) Omeprazole (40 mg) is superior to ranitidine in short-term treatment of reflux esophagitis. Dig Dis Sci 33:523-529

29. Arens MJ, Dent J (1993) Acid pump blockers: what are their current therapeutic role? Bailliéres Clin Gastroenterol 7:95-128

30. Glise H (1989) Healing, relapse rates and prophylaxis of reflux esophagitis. Scand J Gastroenterol 24:57-64

31. Schindlebeck NE, Klauser AG, Berghammer G, Londong WW, Muller-Lissner SA

(1992) Three years follow-up of patients with gastroesophageal reflux disease. Gut 33:1016-1019

32. McDougall NI, Johnston BT, Kee F, Collins JSA, McFarland RJ, Love AHG (1996) Natural history of reflux esophagitis: a 10 year follow up of its effect on patient symptomatology and quality of life. Gut 38:481-486

33. Hillman AL, Bloom B, Frendrick AM (1992) Cost and quality effects of alternative treatments for persistent gastroesophageal reflux disease. Arch Intern Med 152:1467-1472

34. Howden CW, Castell DO, Cohen S, Freston JW, Orlando RC, Robinson M (1995) The rationale for continuous maintenance treatment of reflux esophagitis. Arch Intern Med 155:1465-1471

35. Richter JE (1992) Surgery for reflux disease: reflections of a gastroenterologist. N Engl J Med 326:825-827

36. Walker SJ, Baxter ST, Morris AI, Sutton R (1997) Review article: controversy in the therapy of gastroesophageal reflux disease. Long term proton pump inhibition or laparoscopic anti-reflux surgery? Aliment Pharmacol Ther 11:249-260

37. Peters JH, DeMeester TR (1993) The gastroesophageal reflux. Surg Clin North Am 73:1119-1144

38. Graham DL, Patterson DJ (1983) Double blind comparison of liquid antacid and placebo in the treatment of symptomatic reflux esophagitis. Dig Dis Sci 28:559-566

39. Garnett WR (1993) Efficacy, safety and cost issues in managing patients with gastroesophageal reflux disease. Am J Hosp Pharm 50(Suppl 1):S11-S18

40. Ramirez B, Richter JE (1993) Review article: promotility drugs in the treatment of gastroesophageal reflux disease. Aliment Pharmacol Ther 7:5-20

41. Heitman P, Moler N (1970) The effect of metoclopramide on the gastroesophageal junctional zone and distal esophagus in man. Scand J Gastroenterol 5:620-626

42. Fink SM, Lange RC, McCallum RW (1983) Effect of metoclopramide on normal and delayed gastric emptying in gastroesophageal reflux patients. Dig Dis Sci 28:1057-1061

43. McCallum RW, Ippolitti AF, Cooney C, Sturdevant RA (1977) Controlled trial of metoclopramide in symptomatic gastroesophageal reflux. N Engl J Med 296:354-357

44. Bright-Asare P, El-Bassoussi M (1980) Cimetidine, metoclopramide or placebo in the treatment of symptomatic gastroesophageal reflux. J Clin Gastroenterol 2:149-156

45. McCallum RW, Fink SM, Winnan GR, Avella J, Callahan C (1984) Metoclopramide in gastroesophageal reflux disease: rationale for its use and results of a double-blind trial. Am J Gastroenterol 79:165-172

46. Bron B, Massih L (1980) Domperidone: a drug with powerful action on the lower esophageal sphincter pressure. Digestion 20:375-378

47. Missale G, Missale C, Sigale S, Cestar R, Merno M, Lojacono L, Spano P (1990) Evidence for the presence of both D-1 and D-2 dopamine receptors in human esophagus. Life Sci 47:447-455

48. VanNeuten JM, Schuurkes JAJ (1986) Pharmacodynamics of cisapride, a prokinetic agent with indirect cholinergic properties. Digestion 34:137

49. Gilbert RJ, Dodds WJ, Kahrilas PJ, et al (1987) Effect of cisapride, a new prokinetic agent, in esophageal motor dysfunction. Dig Dis Sci 32:1331-1336

50. Ramirez B, Richter JE (1993) Review article: promotility drugs in the treatment of gastroesophageal reflux disease. Aliment Pharmacol Ther 7:5-20

51. Cooke HJ, Carey HV (1984) The effects of cisapride on serotonin-evoked mucosal response in guinea pig ileum. Eur J Pharmacol 98:147-148

52. Crampton JR, Gibbons LC, Rees WDW (1987) Effects of sucralfate on gastroduodenal bicarbonate and prostaglandin E_2 metabolism. Am J Med 3:83-92

53. Nexo E, Poulsen SS (1987) Does epidermal growth factor play a role in the action of sucralfate? Scand J Gastroenterol 22(Suppl 127):45-49
54. Jensen SL, Jensen PF (1992) Role of sucralfate in peptic disease. Dig Dis Sci 10:153-161
55. McCarthy DM (1991) Sucralfate. N Engl J Med 325:1017-1025
56. Bernardo DE, Lancaster SM, Strickland ID (1975) A double-blind controlled trial of Gaviscon in the patients with symptomatic gastroesophageal reflux. Curr Med Res Opin 3:338-390
57. Graham DY, Lancer F, Dorsch BR (1977) Symptomatic reflux esophagitis: a double blind controlled comparison of antacids and alginate. Curr Ther Res 22:653
58. McHardy G (1978) A multicenter randomized clinical trial of Gaviscon in reflux esophagitis. South Med J 71:16-21
59. Meuwissen SG, Klinkenberg-Knol EC (1988) Treatment of reflux esophagitis with H_2 receptor antagonists. Scand J Gastroenterol 23:201-213
60. Koelz HR (1989) Treatment of reflux esophagitis with H_2 blockers, antacid and prokinetic drugs. Scand J Gastroenterol 156:25-36
61. Colin Jones DG (1989) Histamine H_2 receptor antagonists in gastroesophageal reflux. Gut 30:1305-1308
62. Feldman M, Burton ME (1990) Histamine$_2$-receptor antagonists: standard therapy for acid-peptic diseases. N Engl J Med 323:1672-1680 (part one)/1749-1755 (part two)
63. Lipsy RJ, Fennerty B, Fagan TC (1990) Clinical review of histamine$_2$-receptor antagonists. Arch Intern Med 150:745-751
64. Somogyi A, Muirhead M (1988) Pharmacokinetic interactions of cimetidine. Clin Pharmacokinet 12:321-366
65. Hixson LJ, Kelley CL, Jones WN, Tuohy CD (1992) Current trends in the pharmacology for gastroesophageal reflux disease. Arch Intern Med 152:717-723
66. Chiba N, de Cara CJ, Wilkinson JM, Hunt RH (1997) Speed of healing and symptom relief in grade II to IV gastro-oesophageal reflux disease: a meta-analysis. Gastroenterology 112:1798-1810
67. Lindberg P, Brandstrom A, Wallmark B, Manson H, Rikner L, Hoffmann KJ (1990) Omeprazole: the first proton pump inhibitor. Med Res Rev 10:1-54
68. Nagaya H, Satoh H, Kubo K, Maki Y (1989) Possible mechanism for the inhibition of gastric (H^+/K^+) adenosine triphosphate by the proton pump inhibitor AG-1749. J Pharmacol Exp Ther 248:799-805
69. Tolman KG, Sanders SW, Bucli KR (1994) Gastric pH levels after 15 mg and 30 mg of lansoprazole and 20 mg of omeprazole. Gastroenterology 106:A197
70. Hatlebakk JG, Berstad A, Carling L, Svedberg LE, Unge P, Ekstrom P (1993) Lansoprazole vs omeprazole in short term treatment of reflux esophagitis. Results of a Scandinavian multicentre trial. Scand J Gastroenterol 28:224-228
71. Castell DO, Richter JE, Robinson M, Sontag S (1995) Large trial compares lansoprazole to omeprazole. Gastroenterology 108(Suppl 4):A67
72. Larsson H, Hakanson R, Mattsson H, et al (1988) Omeprazole: its influence on gastric acid secretion, gastrin and ECL cells. Toxicol Pathol 16:267-272
73. Ekman L, Hansson E, Havu N, Carlsson E, Lundberg C (1987) Toxicological studies on omeprazole. Scand J Gastroenterol 20(Suppl 108):53-69
74. Hetzel DJ, Dent J, Reed WD, et al (1988) Healing and relapse of severe peptic esophagitis after treatment with omeprazole. Gastroenterology 95:903-912
75. Brunner G, Creutzfeldt W, Harke U, et al (1989) Efficacy and safety of long term treatment with omeprazole in patients with acid related diseases resistant to ranitidine. Scand J Gastroenterol 3(Suppl A):72-76

76. McClay RF (1992) Implication of a review of omeprazole and management strategies for peptic disease. Hepatogastroenterology 39:90-91
77. Kuipers EJ, Uyterlinde AM, Pena AS, et al (1995) Long-term sequelae of *Helicobacter pylori* gastritis. Lancet 345:1525-1528
78. Kuipers EJ, Lundell L, Klinkenberg-Knol EC, et al (1996) Atrophic gastritis and *Helicobacter pylori* infection in patients with reflux esophagitis treated with omeprazole or fundoplication. N Engl J Med 334:1018-1022
79. Labenz J, Malfertheiner P (1997) *Helicobacter pylori* in gastroesophageal reflux disease: causal agent, independent or protective factor? Gut 41:277-280
80. Meyer UA (1996) Metabolic interactions of the proton pump inhibitors lansoprazole, omeprazole and pantoprazole with others drugs. Eur J Gastroenterol Hepatol 8(Suppl 1):S21-S25
81. Kromer W, Postius S, Riedel R, et al (1990) BY1023/SK&F 96022 INN pantoprazole, a novel gastric proton pump inhibitor potently inhibits acid secretion but lacks relevant cytocrome P450 interactions. J Pharmacol Exp Ther 254:129-135
82. Kohl B, Sturm E, Senn-Bilfinger J, et al (1992) (H^+/K^+)-ATPase inhibiting 2-(2-pyridyl-methyl sulphinyl) benzimidazoles. A novel series of dimethoxy pyridyl-substituted inhibitors with enhanced selectivity: the selection of pantoprazole as a clinical candidate. J Med Chem 35:1094-1097
83. Huber R, Kohl B, Sachs G, et al (1995) Review article: the continuing development of proton pump inhibitors with particular reference to pantoprazole. Aliment Pharmacol Ther 9:363-378
84. Beil W, Staar U, Sewing KF (1992) Pantoprazole: a novel H^+/K^+ ATPase inhibitor with an improved pH stability. Eur J Pharmacol 218:265-271
85. Shin JM, Besançon M, Prinz C, et al (1994) Continuing development of acid pump inhibitors: site of action of pantoprazole. Aliment Pharmacol Ther 8(Suppl 1):11-23
86. Steinijans VW, Huber R, Hartmann M, Zech K, Bliesath H, Wurst W, et al (1996) Lack of pantoprazole drug interactions in man: an updated review. Int J Clin Pharmacol Ther 34:243-262
87. Hartmann M, Bliesath H, Zech K, Koch H, Steinijans VW, Wurst W, et al (1995) Pantoprazole does not influence CYP1A2 activity in man. Gastroenterology 108(Suppl 4):A109
88. Corinaldesi R, Valentino M, Belaïche J, Colin R, Gerdof M, Maier C (1995) Pantoprazole and omeprazole in the treatment of reflux esophagitis: a European multicentric study. Aliment Pharmacol Ther 9:667-671
89. Vicari F, Belin J, Marek L (1998) Pantoprazole 40 mg vs. omeprazole 20 mg in the treatment of reflux esophagitis: results of a French multicentric double-blind comparative trial. In: Abstract book, World Congress of Gastroenterology, 6-11 September, Vienna, p 487
90. Hotz J, Brandstäter G, Fumagalli I (1996) Comparative study of pantoprazole vs. omeprazole used in acute treatment of reflux esophagitis. Gut 39(Suppl 3):A34
91. Mössner J, Koop H, Porst H, Wübbolding H, Schneider A, Maier C (1997) A one year study on efficacy and safety of pantoprazole on prevention of relapse of reflux esophagitis. Aliment Pharmacol Ther 11:1087-1092
92. Van Rensburg CJ, Honiball PJ, De K, Grundling H, van Zyl JH, Spies SK, et al (1997) Long-term (2 years) efficacy and safety of pantoprazole 40 mg on the prevention of reflux esophagitis relapse. Gut 41(Suppl 3):P728
93. Plein K, Hotz J, Wurzer H, Fumagalli I, Tenor H, Schneider A (1998) Prevention of relapse in gastroesophageal reflux disease (GERD). A randomized, double-blind, long-term, multi-centre study using 20 mg or 40 mg of pantoprazole. In: Abstract

book, World Congress of Gastroenterology, 6-11 September, Vienna, p 483

94. Galmiche JP, Janssens J (1995) The pathophysiology of gastroesophageal reflux disease: an overview. Scand J Gastroenterol 30(Suppl 211):7-18

95. Boeckxstaens GE, Tytgat GNJ (1996) Pathophysiology, diagnosis and treatment of gastroesophageal reflux disease. Curr Opin Gastroenterol 12:365-372

96. Timmer R, Breumelhof R, Nadorp JHSM, Smout AJPM (1993) Recent advances in the pathophysiology of gastroesophageal reflux disease. Eur J Gastroenterol Hepatol 5:485-491

97. Vicari J, Falk GW, Richter JE (1997) *Helicobacter pylori* and acid peptic disorders: is it conceivable? Am J Gastroenterol 92:1097-1102

98. de Koster E, Kuipers EJ (1997) Reflux and *Helicobacter pylori*. Curr Opin Gastroenterol 13:43-47

99. Werdmuller BFM, Loffeld RJLF (1997) *Helicobacter pylori* infection has no role in the pathogenesis of reflux esophagitis. Dig Dis Sci 42:103-105

100. Janssens J, Sifrim D (1995) Spontaneous transient lower esophageal sphincter relaxations: a target for treatment of gastroesophageal reflux disease. Gastroenterology 109:1703-1706

The Role of Respiratory Drugs in Gastroesophageal Reflux

M. Cazzola[1], S. Centanni[2], M.G. Matera[1], and R.W. Dal Negro

Introduction

Most adult asthmatics have abnormal gastroesophageal reflux manifested by increased reflux frequency, delayed acid clearance during the day and night, and diminished lower oesophageal sphincter pressure; this happens regardless of the use of bronchodilator therapy [1]. Epidemiological evidence for the association between gastroesophageal reflux and asthma suggests that, quite apart from the need for bronchodilators, about three-fourths of asthmatics have acid gastroesophageal reflux, increased frequency of reflux episodes or heartburn, and 40% have reflux oesophagitis [2].

One or more of three possible relationships may exist between asthma and gastroesophageal reflux: (1) both may occur in the same patient and be unrelated; (2) the physiologic effects of airway obstruction and measures used in an attempt to reverse it may worsen gastroesophageal reflux; or (3) the reflux of gastric contents may worsen or precipitate airway obstruction [3]. Flattening of the diaphragm associated with air trapping during bronchoconstriction may reduce the competency of the lower oesophageal sphincter [4]. Indeed, the pressure in the lower oesophageal sphincter of asthmatics is significantly lower than that of controls when measured manometrically [1, 5]. With acute exacerbation, asthma results in a state of more negative intrathoracic pressure versus more positive intra-abdominal pressure, exaggerating the gradient favouring gastroesophageal reflux [6]. For this reason it has been suggested that treatment of asthma might lessen the occurrence of gastroesophageal reflux [7]. Conversely, it is also possible that attempts at medical management of asthma worsen gastroesophageal reflux. In fact, several studies suggest an association between gastroesophageal reflux and treatments with antiasthmatic drugs. Nevertheless, many investigators refute the possibility of such an effect. For example, it is well known that asthmatics have significant gastroesophageal

[1]Clinical Pharmacology Unit and Respiratory Pharmacology Centre, Salvatore Maugeri Foundation, IRCCS, Rehabilitation Institute, Veruno (Novara), Italy; [2]Institute of Respiratory Diseases, University of Milan, IRCCS Ospedale Maggiore, Milan, Italy; [3]Lung Department, Bussolengo General Hospital, Bussolengo (Verona), Italy

reflux when asleep and after meals that continues beyond the post-prandial period to the next meal. In addition, asthma patients receiving bronchodilators experience gastroesophageal reflux patterns after eating, in the nonprandial period and when asleep, which are similar to those of asthmatics not receiving bronchodilators [3].

However, a possibility that bronchodilators might influence gastro-esophageal reflux exists. We must emphasise that there are important interactions between the oesophagus and the lower respiratory tract. These occur because of their physical proximity and functional activities. Malfunction or lack of co-ordination between these organs leads to gastroesophageal reflux [9]. Tonic contraction of the lower oesophageal sphincter is believed to be the principal mechanism preventing gastroesophageal reflux. Virtually all reflux episodes occur when lower oesophageal sphincter pressure is absent. For this reason, all drugs which inhibit oesophageal motor function may potentially induce gastroesophageal reflux [10].

Neuronal Control of Oesophageal Function

Oesophageal peristalsis and sphincter function are controlled by the autonomic nervous system, with contributions from parasympathetic, sympathetic, and enteric divisions [11]. Vagal stimulation evokes lower oesophageal sphincter relaxation via activation of established cholinergic and non-adrenergic non-cholinergic (NANC) mechanisms and other unidentified mechanisms. In any case, nitric oxide (NO) plays an important role as a neurotransmitter in NANC inhibitory nerves of the human lower oesophageal sphincter [12]. Splanchnic stimulation activates adrenergic neurones probably via nicotinic and non-nicotinic ganglionic mechanisms, which in turn elicit β-adrenergic inhibitory effects on the lower oesophageal sphincter [13].

Muscarinic participation in vagally induced lower oesophageal sphincter relaxation exhibits two functional receptor subtypes: (1) M_1 receptors that determine lower oesophageal sphincter relaxation latency and are antagonised by pirenzepine (a selective muscarinic M_1 antagonist) or atropine (a nonselective muscarinic antagonist), and (2) M_3 receptors that contribute to the magnitude of lower oesophageal sphincter relaxation and are antagonised by atropine, but not by pirenzepine or 4-DAMP (a selective muscarinic M_2 antagonist) [14]. In particular, lower oesophageal sphincter contraction is mediated through M_3 receptors, a pertussis toxin-insensitive G9-G11 protein, activation of phospholipase C (PLC), inositol 1,4,5,-trisphosphate (IP3) formation and the release of intracellular Ca^{2+} [15].

Experimental data suggest the presence of β_1- as well as β_2-adrenoceptors on circular muscle from the human oesophagogastric junction; both receptors mediate inhibition of active resting tension [16]. The presence of specific β-receptors in the human lower oesophageal sphincter has been confirmed by Thorpe [17]. This author showed that intravenously administered propranolol induced a significant increase in sphincter pressure in human volunteers. Recently, it has been documented that β_3-adrenoceptor isotypes mediate isopranaline-induced relaxation of lower oesophageal sphincter, at least in rat. This activation is not linked to either ATPase-dependent or Ca^{2+}-dependent K^+ channels or to NO release [18].

It is interesting to highlight that intra-oesophageal acid caused substance P release from extrinsic afferent nerve endings and activated local inhibitory pathways to the lower oesophageal sphincter via neurokinin-1 (NK-1) receptors [19]. Substance P also caused activation of myenteric NANC inhibitory neurones and sympathetic neurones [13].

Bronchodilators and Lower Oesophageal Sphincter Activity

Both β-agonists and methylxanthines inhibit active resting tension of isolated muscle strips from the human oesophageal-gastric junction [16]. In effect, all bronchodilators (anticholinergic, theophylline, β_2-agonists) promote acid production or reduce the lower oesophageal sphincter time. Unfortunately, some persons are not aware of this problem before bronchodilator treatment becomes more aggressive.

Methylxanthines

A possible role of methylxanthines in the high incidence of gastroesophageal reflux in patients with asthma has been documented. In fact, these agents at therapeutic serum levels increase gastric secretion and decrease lower oesophageal pressure that, in turn, possibly increase gastroesophageal reflux in normal adults [20].

Vandenplas and colleagues [21] examined the influence of xanthines on gastroesophageal reflux in infants at risk for sudden infant death syndrome. Thirty babies were tested for gastroesophageal reflux before and during caffeine treatment. Eighteen were studied under the same conditions while undergoing theophylline treatment. All results of pH monitoring before treatment were within normal ranges. Episodes of gastroesophageal reflux increased significantly in about 50% of the group treated with caffeine and in 66% of the group treated with theophylline. These results were independent of plasma xanthine concentrations and of the efficacy of the drug. In addition, an increase was noted for the number of episodes of gastroesophageal reflux in 24 hours and for the time that pH was less than 4. Ekström and Tibbling [22] showed that the normal maintenance dose of theophylline caused a significant increase in total reflux time and reflux symptoms, but did not worsen the asthma in 25 patients with moderate to severe asthma and a history of respiratory symptoms aggravated by reflux. Patients with subtherapeutic serum levels showed significant improvement in lung function while those with therapeutic serum levels did not. Hervé and colleagues [23] confirmed that treatment with theophylline could constitute a risk factor for gastroesophageal reflux in chronic asthma. In particular, they observed that the only predictive factor for the presence of gastroesophageal reflux was the dosage of theophylline whose average dose was higher in cases of gastroesophageal reflux. On the other hand, the severity of gastroesophageal reflux, assessed as the percentage of the total time passed with a pH below 4, also correlated with the longevity of the disease.

Unfortunately, other studies refute a role for methylxanthines in gastroesophageal reflux. Johannesson and colleagues [24] documented that adenosine antagonism regulates gastric secretion, but not lower oesophageal sphincter pressure. This difference is likely since enprophylline does not regulate gastric secretion, while both theophylline and enprophylline are able to relax the sphincter, probably from phosphodiesterase inhibition. Nonetheless, Hubert and colleagues [25] failed to demonstrate any adverse effect of a slow-release theophylline preparation on gastroesophageal reflux in patients with asthma. Moreover, Berquist and colleagues [26] proved that in chronic asthmatic children, standard oral theophylline therapy did not adversely affect silent gastroesophageal reflux. It may be speculated that the decrease of lower oesophageal sphincter pressure may be counterbalanced by the bronchodilator effect of this drug [25].

β_2-Agonists

When given intravenously or orally, β-agonists are associated with a reduction of lower oesophageal sphincter tone in healthy subjects [27]. Unfortunately, there are no truly comparable data suggesting that systemic application of β_2-agonists is also associated with an increased number of reflux events during 24-hour pH monitoring (pH-metry). Both oral carbuterol [28] and parenteral terbutaline [29] significantly decreased lower oesophageal sphincter pressure. However, several studies did not demonstrate an adverse effect of oral β-agonists on the frequency of gastroesophageal reflux. In fact, metaproterenol sulfate did not induce a significant increase in gastroesophageal reflux in asthmatic children or normal adults [26]. Moreover, 4 mg salbutamol by mouth did not affect oesophageal function [30].

The effect of inhaled bronchodilators on gastroesophageal reflux is less clear. It is well known that inhalation of β_2-adrenergic drugs results in less systemic side effects than does oral application [31]. This also may apply to oesophageal side effects. In fact, patients with gastroesophageal reflux disease who require bronchodilator therapy for obstructive lung disease apparently have less reflux with inhaled agents. For example, Schindlbeck and colleagues [32] investigated the influence of inhalation of salbutamol on oesophageal motor function and gastroesophageal reflux in ten healthy volunteers. Inhalation decreased neither lower oesophageal sphincter pressure nor oesophageal peristaltic amplitudes. Furthermore, Ruzkowski and colleagues [33] compared the severity of gastroesophageal reflux in patients with documented gastroesophageal reflux disease and obstructive lung disease while they were taking inhaled salbutamol or oral theophylline. Patients taking salbutamol had 40% less total time with pH < 4.0 than those with theophylline and less gastroesophageal reflux. A lower systemic level of these drugs after inhalation compared with oral or intravenous application is the most likely reason for less reflux. However, a questionnaire-based, cross-sectional analytic survey demonstrated a greater prevalence of gastroesophageal reflux symptoms in asthmatic patients [34]. Moreover, gastroesophageal reflux symptoms were associated with increased β-agonist inhaler use.

Anticholinergics

The lower oesophageal sphincter has two components, one of which is acid-sensitive and both of which are atropine-sensitive [35]. The presence of these components justifies why 0.05-0.06 mg atropine i.v. injection decreases lower oesophageal sphincter pressure [36, 37]. As a result, anticholinergic agents are widely believed to exacerbate gastroesophageal reflux. However, in dogs, reflux that occurs during atropine-induced ablation of lower oesophageal sphincter pressure is intermittent and also associated with inhibition of the crural diaphragm, suggesting that the latter is a prerequisite for reflux [38].

Aggestrup and Jensen [39] showed that intravenously administered pirenzepine and atropine both inhibited basal lower oesophageal sphincter pressure and oesophageal peristalsis in healthy volunteers, regardless of the employed doses. This effect should be important in patients with asthma in whom reflux may contribute to bronchospasm. However, reflux due to atropine has not been shown to be associated with untoward effects on the airways [40]. In particular, atropine-induced lower oesophageal sphincter pressure reduction did not predispose to reflux in normal healthy subjects [41]. The reason for the reduction in the frequency of reflux was a decrease in the frequency of transient lower oesophageal sphincter relaxation by atropine. When the lower oesophageal sphincter pressure is low, the crural diaphragm may act as an important antireflux barrier [41]. This finding might explain why Mittal and colleagues [42] have recently documented that atropine (15 μg/kg intravenous bolus and 4 μg/kg h as a maintenance dose) reduces the frequency of spontaneous reflux in healthy subjects. It has also been shown that atropine inhibits reflux in patients with reflux disease largely by inhibition of lower oesophageal sphincter relaxations and swallow-induced lower oesophageal sphincter relaxation [43].

The therapeutic potential for anticholinergic agents in reducing the frequency of reflux and of transient lower oesophageal sphincter relaxation awaits investigation. Nowadays, there is no evidence In the literature that inhaled anticholinergics influence gastroesophageal reflux. Both ipratropium bromide and oxitropium bromide are quaternary ammonium muscarinic receptor antagonists. Less than 1% of an inhaled dose of these agents is absorbed systematically. As with most drugs administered by aerosol, about 90% of a dose is swallowed. However, their quaternary structure limits absorption through the mucous membrane of the respiratory and gastrointestinal tracts; therefore, most of the drug is not absorbed and appears in the faeces [44]. Because of this pharmacokinetic behaviour, inhaled anticholinergics might not interfere with lower oesophageal sphincter activity.

Other Antiasthmatic Medications

The fact that intra-oesophageal acid releases tachykinins, probably substance P, from the sensory neurones and results in plasma extravasation in the airways [45] raises the question if antiasthmatic drugs which are thought to act via inhibition of substance P release (e.g. nedocromil sodium [46] and azelastine [47]) may beneficially influence gastroesophageal reflux-induced asthma. It has been suggested that oesophageal shortening associated with acute acid-induced oesophageal injury is dependent on mast cell-derived mediators. In fact, pre-treatment with disodium cromoglycate in doses sufficient to attenuate the acid-induced mucosal histamine release, blocks acid perfusion-induced oesophageal shortening, but not electrical field stimulation-induced oesophageal shortening [48]. Alternatively since substance P activates local inhibitory pathways to the lower oesophageal sphincter [49], it is possible that tachykinin receptor antagonists may have a role. These are important points because communication between the oesophagus and airway likely involves a local axon reflex [50]. Unfortunately, these questions are still without an answer.

References

1. Sontag SJ, O'Connell S, Khandelwal S, Miller T, Nemchausky B, Schnell TG, Serlovsky R (1990) Most asthmatics have gastroesophageal reflux with or without bronchodilator therapy. Gastroenterology 99:613-620
2. Sontag SJ (1997) Gastroesophageal reflux and asthma. Am J Med 1093:84S-90S
3. Sontag SJ, O'Connell S, Khandelwal S, Miller T, Nemchausky B, Schnell TG, Serlovsky R (1990) Effect of positions, eating, and bronchodilators on gastroesophageal reflux in asthmatics. Dig Dis Sci 35:849-856
4. Simpson WG (1995) Gastroesophageal reflux disease and asthma. Diagnosis and management. Arch Intern Med 155:798-803
5. Harding SM, Richter JE (1992) Gatroesophageal reflux disease and asthma. Semin Gastrointest Dis 3:130-150
6. Harper PC, Bergner A, Kaye MD (1987) Antireflux treatment for asthma: improvement in patients with associated gastroesophageal reflux. Arch Intern Med 147:56-60
7. Homes PW, Campbell AM, Barter CE (1978) Changes of lung volumes and mechanics in asthma and normal subjects. Thorax 33:394-400
8. Singh V, Jain NK (1983) Asthma as a cause for, rather than a result of, gastroesophageal reflux. J Asthma 20:241
9. Mansfield LE (1995) Associations and interactions between the esophagus and the lower respiratory tract. Pediatr Pulmonol 11(Suppl):53-54
10. Dodds WJ, Dent J Hogan WJ, Helm JF, Hauser RH, Patel GK, Egide MS (1982) Mechanisms of gastroesophageal reflux in patients with reflux esophagitis. N Engl J Med 307:1547-1552

11. Richards WG, Sugarbaker DJ (1995) Neuronal control of esophageal function. Chest Surg Clin N Am 5:157-171

12. Tomita R, Kurosu Y, Munakata K (1997) Relationship between nitric oxide and non-adrenergic non-cholinergic inhibitory nerves in human lower esophageal sphincter. J Gastroenterol 32:1-5

13. Blackshaw LA, Haupt JA, Omari T, Dent J (1997) Vagal and sympathetic influences on the ferret lower oesophageal sphincter. J Auton Nerv Syst 66:179-188

14. Gilbert RJ, Dodds WJ (1987) Subtypes of muscarinic receptors in vagal inhibitory pathway to the lower esophageal sphincter of the opossum. Dig Dis Sci 32:1130-1135

15. Sohn UD, Harnett KM, De Petris G, Behar J, Biancani P (1993) Distinct muscarinic receptors, G proteins and phospholipases in esophageal and lower esophageal sphincter circular muscle. J Pharmacol Exp Ther 267:1205-1214

16. Tottrup A, Forman A, Madsen G, Andersson KE (1990) The actions of some beta-receptor agonists and xanthines on isolated muscle strips from human oesophago-gastric junction. Pharmacol Toxicol 67:340-343

17. Thorpe JA (1980) Effect of propanolol on the lower oesophageal sphincter in man. Curr Med Res Opin 7:91-95

18. Oriowo MA (1997) Beta$_3$-adrenoceptors mediate smooth muscle relaxation in the rat lower esophageal sphincter. J Auton Pharmacol 17:175-182

19. Blackshaw LA, Dent J (1997) Lower oesophageal sphincter responses to noxious oesophageal chemical stimuli in the ferret: involvement of tachykinin receptors. J Auton Nerv Syst 66:189-200

20. Berquist WE, Rachelefsky GS, Kadden M, Siegel SC, Katz RM, Mickey MR, Ament ME (1981) Effect of theophylline on gastroesophageal reflux in normal adults. J Allergy Clin Immunol 67:407-411

21. Vandenplas Y, De Wolf D, Sacre L (1986) The influence of xanthines on gastroesophageal reflux in infants at risk for sudden infant death syndrome. Pediatrics 77:807-810

22. Ekström T, Tibbling L (1988) Influence of theophylline on gastro-oesophageal reflux and asthma. Eur J Clin Pharmacol 35:353-356

23. Hervé P, Escourrou P, Salmeron S, Gandolfo JY, Charley S, Denjean A, Petitpretz P, Simonneau G, Gaultier C, Duroux P (1993) Facteurs de risque de reflux gastro-oesophagien dans l'asthme chronique. Rev Mal Respir 10:527-530

24. Johannesson N, Andersson KE, Joelsson B, Persson CG (1985) Relaxation of lower esophageal sphincter and stimulation of gastric secretion and diuresis by antiasthmatic xanthines. Role for adenosine antagonism. Am Rev Respir Dis 131:26-30

25. Hubert D, Gaudric M, Guerre J, Lockhart A, Marsac J (1988) Effect of theophylline on gastroesophageal reflux in patients with asthma. J Allergy Clin Immunol 81:1168-1174

26. Berquist WE, Rachelesky GS, Rowshan N, Siegel S, Katz R, Welch M (1984) Quantitative gastroesophageal reflux and pulmonary function in asthmatic children and normal adults receiving placebo, theophylline, and metaproterenol sulfate therapy. J Allergy Clin Immunol 73:255-258

27. Zfass AM, Prince R, Allen FN, Farrar JT (1970) Inhibitory beta-adrenergic receptors in the human distal esophagus. Dig Dis 15:303-310

28. Di Marino AJ, Cohen S (1982) Effect of an oral beta-2 adrenergic agonist on lower esophageal sphincter pressure in normals and in patients with achalasia. Dig Dis Sci 27:1063-1066

29. Wong RK, Maydonovitch C, Garcia JE, Johnson LF, Castell DO (1987) The effect of terbutaline sulfate, nitroglycerin, and aminophylline on lower esophageal sphincter

pressure and radionuclide esophageal emptying in patients with achalasia. J Clin Gastroenterol 9:386-389

30. Michoud MC, Ledue T, Proulx F, Perreault S, Du Souich P, Duranceau A, Amyot R (1991) Effect of salbutamol on gastroesophageal reflux in healthy volunteers and patients with asthma. J Allergy Clin Immunol 87:762-767

31. Larsson S, Svedmyr N (1977) Bronchodilating effect and side effects of beta-2-adrenoceptor stimulants by different modes of administration (tablets, metered aerosol, and combinations thereof). Am Rev Respir Dis 116:861-869

32. Schindlbeck NE, Heinrich C, Huber RM, Muller-Lissner SA (1988) Effects of albuterol (salbutamol) on esophageal motility and gastroesophageal reflux in healthy volunteers. JAMA 260:3156-3158

33. Ruzkowski CJ, Sanowski RA, Austin J, Rohwedder JJ, Waring JP (1992) The effects of inhaled salbutamol and oral theophylline on gastroesophageal reflux in patients with gastroesophageal reflux disease and obstructive lung disease. Arch Intern Med 152:783-785

34. Field SK, Underwood M, Brant R, Cowie RL (1996) Prevalence of gastroesophageal reflux symptoms in asthma. Chest 109:316-322

35. McLean TR, Bombeck CT, Nyhus LM (1987) Distinction of lower esophageal sphincter strength from sphincter competence. Am J Surg 153:91-95

36. Cotton BR, Smith G (1981) Comparison of the effects of atropine and glycopyrrolate on lower oesophageal sphincter pressure. Br J Anaesth 53:875-879

37. Opie JC, Chaye H, Steward DJ (1987) Intravenous atropine rapidly reduces lower esophageal sphincter pressure in infants and children. Anesthesiology 67:989-990

38. Martin CJ, Dodds WJ, Liem HH, Dantas RO, Layman RD, Dent J (1992) Diaphragmatic contribution to gastroesophageal competence and reflux in dogs. Am J Physiol 263:G551-G557

39. Aggestrup S, Jensen SL (1991) Effects of pirenzerpine and atropine on basal lower esophageal pressure and gastric acid secretion in man: a placebo-controlled randomized study. Dig Dis 9:360-364

40. Gross NJ (1993) Safety and side-effects of anticholinergic bronchodilators. In: Gross NJ (ed) Anticholinergic therapy in obstructive airways disease. Franklin Scientific, London, pp 116-127

41. Mittal RK, Holloway R, Dent J (1995) Effect of atropine on the frequency of reflux and transient lower esophageal sphincter relaxation in normal subjects. Gastroenterology 109:1547-1554

42. Mittal RK, Chiareli C, Liu J, Holloway R, Dixon W Jr (1997) Atropine inhibits gastric distension and pharyngeal receptor mediated lower oesophageal sphincter relaxation. Gut 41:285-290

43. Lidums I, Checklin H, Mittal RK, Holloway RH (1998) Effect of atropine on gastro-oesophageal reflux and transient lower oesophageal sphincter relaxation in patients with gastro-oesophageal reflux disease. Gut 43:12-16

44. Brown JH, Taylor P (1996) Muscarinic receptor agonists and antagonists. In: Hardman JG, Limbird LE, Milinoff PB, Euddon RW, Goodman Gilman A (eds) Goodman & Gilman's the pharmacological basis of therapeutics, 9th edn. McGraw-Hill, New York, pp 141-160

45. Hamamoto J, Kohrogi H, Kawano O, Iwagoe H, Fujii K, Hirata N, Ando M (1997) Esophageal stimulation by hydrochloric acid causes neurogenic inflammation in the airways of guinea pigs. J Appl Physiol 82:738-745

46. Chung KF (1996) Effects of nedocromil sodium on airway neurogenic mechanisms. J Allergy Clin Immunol 98:S112-S116

47. Nieber K, Baumgarten C, Rathsack R, Furkert J, Laake E, Muller S, Kunkel G (1993)

Effect of azelastine on substance P content in bronchoalveolar and nasal lavage fluids of patients with allergic asthma. Clin Exp Allergy 23:69-71
48. Paterson WG (1998) Role of most cell-derived mediators in acid-induced shortening of the esophagus. Am J Physiol 274:G385-G388
49. Blachshaw LA, Dent J (1988) Lower oesophageal sphincter responses to noxious oesophageal chemical stimuli in the ferret: involvment of tachykinin receptors. J Autonom Nerv Syst 13:189-200
50. Bechard D, Schubert M (1998) Gatroesophageal reflux-induced asthma: new insights. Gastroenterology 114:894-850

Made in the USA
Monee, IL
07 July 2026

56552209R00118

Springer-Verlag Italia Srl.